# DISEASES OF FISHES

Edited by
DR. STANISLAS F. SNIESZKO
and
DR. HERBERT R. AXELROD

## Book 6:
## FUNGAL DISEASES OF FISHES

This is the sixth book in the series dealing with diseases of fishes.

by
**Gordon A. Neish**
Mycology Section,
Biosystematics Research Institute,
Agriculture Canada
Ottawa, Canada K1A OC6

and
**Gilbert C. Hughes**
Department of Botany and
Institute of Oceanography
University of British Columbia
Vancouver, Canada V6T 1W5

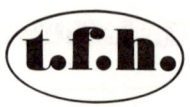

ISBN 0-87666-504-0

© 1980 by T.F.H Publications, Inc., Ltd.

Distributed in the U.S. by T.F.H. Publications, Inc., 211 West Sylvania Avenue, PO Box 427, Neptune, NJ 07753; in England by T.F.H. (Gt. Britain) Ltd., 13 Nutley Lane, Reigate, Surrey; in Canada to the book store and library trade by Beaverbooks Ltd., 150 Lesmill Road, Don Mills, Ontario M38 2T5, Canada; in Canada to the pet trade by Rolf C. Hagen Ltd., 3225 Sartelon Street, Montreal 382, Quebec; in Southeast Asia by Y.W. Ong, 9 Lorong 36 Geylang, Singapore 14; in Australia and the South Pacific by Pet Imports Pty. Ltd., P.O. Box 149, Brookvale 2100, N.S.W. Australia; in South Africa by Valid Agencies, P.O. Box 51901, Randburg 2125 South Africa. Published by T.F.H. Publications, Inc., Ltd, the British Crown Colony of Hong Kong.

# CONTENTS

**ACKNOWLEDGMENTS** .................................. 5
**INTRODUCTION** ...................................... 7
**OOMYCETES** ......................................... 9
   MORPHOLOGY AND TAXONOMY ................. 9
   INVESTIGATIONS OF SAPROLEGNIOSIS:
   A BRIEF HISTORICAL OUTLINE ................ 19
   PATHOLOGY ....................................... 42
      Isolation and Culture of the Parasite ............... 42
      Gross Pathology ................................ 43
      Histopathology ................................. 45
   PREVENTION AND TREATMENT ................ 47
***BRANCHIOMYCES*** .................................... 50
   SYSTEMATICS, PATHOLOGY, AND
   EPIZOOTIOLOGY ................................ 50
   PREVENTION AND TREATMENT ................ 59
***ICHTHYOPHONUS*** ................................... 61
   SYSTEMATICS .................................... 61
   *ICHTHYOPHONUS HOFERI*: MORPHOLOGY
   AND DEVELOPMENT .......................... 64
   *ICHTHYOPHONUS HOFERI*: PATHOLOGY
   AND EPIZOOTIOLOGY ........................ 86
   PREVENTION AND TREATMENT ............... 100
**FUNGI IMPERFECTI** ................................. 101
   BLASTOMYCETES ................................ 101
   HYPHOMYCETES ................................. 104
      *Aureobasidium* ................................. 105
      *Exophiala* ..................................... 106
      *Fusarium culmorum* ........................... 111
      *Ochroconis* .................................... 111
         *Ochroconis humicola* ..................... 112
         *Ochroconis tshawytschae* ................. 115
      *Verticillium piscis* ............................. 116

    COELOMYCETES ............................... 116
**ASCOMYCETES** .................................... **120**
***DERMOCYSTIDIUM*** .............................. **122**
    INTRODUCTION ............................. 122
    EPIZOOTIOLOGY ............................ 123
    PATHOLOGY ................................ 124
    PREVENTION AND TREATMENT ............... 126
**References** ......................................... **129**
**Index** ............................................... **155**

# Acknowledgments

Although we must accept full responsibility for errors of fact or interpretation, it would not have been possible to complete this book without the support and cooperation of friends and colleagues who provided illustrations, manuscripts in advance of publication, and advice in their areas of expertise. In particular we wish to thank Libero Ajello, Gordon R. Bell, Vicky S. Blazer, Ivan Borroni, Trevor P.T. Evelyn. Gianluigi Giussani, Roger Goos, Ettore Grimaldi, S.J. Hughes, T.W. Johnson, Bob Kabata, Douglas S. King, Ross F. Nigrelli, Nicole Nolard-Tintigner, Raffaele Peduzzi, Frank O. Perkins, H.-H. Reichenbach-Klinke, Ronald J. Roberts, Richard E. Wolke, and William T. Yasutake. Any success this book might have as a positive contribution to veterinary mycology will in large part be because of their willingness to assist in so many ways in its preparation.

We are also indebted to Laure Wilson Neish for her invaluable assistance in the final preparation of the manuscript and to the librarians at the University of British Columbia who gave so much of their time and talent to locating the reference materials on which this book is based. Permission to reproduce previously published illustrative materials was kindly granted by Academic Press, Inc., Acta Zoologica et Pathologica Antverpiensia, Journal of Fish Biology, Journal of the Fisheries Research Board of Canada, Journal of Pathology, Memorie del'Istituto Italiano di Idrobiologia, and the University of Wisconsin Press. Their assistance is gratefully acknowledged.

Our thanks to Drs. S.F. Snieszko and H.R. Axelrod, editors of this series of textbooks, for their helpful advice, interest, and encouragement throughout production of this book.

Work from the University of British Columbia reported here was supported by grants from the Fisheries Research Board of Canada and the National Research Council of Canada (Grant A-2561) to GCH and by an NRC Fellowship to GAN. Preparation of this book was also made possible by support from the National Research Council of Canada through Grant A-2561.

# Introduction

This book is written with the object of providing fisheries biologists, fish pathologists, and mycologists with an up-to-date treatment of what is known of fungal diseases of fishes. The literature dealing with these diseases is extensive, going back more than two hundred years, and is scattered through a wide variety of journals, books, theses, and reports written in a number of languages. In addition, much of the literature is generally difficult to obtain in any except the largest research libraries. We have attempted here to survey this literature and to discuss these fungal diseases of fishes from the viewpoint of mycologists with an interest in fish pathology.

During the preparation of this volume we were struck by the fact that although research on mycoses of fishes has increased tremendously in the past decade, answers to many of the fundamental mycological questions are still missing. So much of the recent research has tended to generate new problems instead of answering old questions! For example, the systematic position of *Branchiomyces* is still uncertain and whether or not it exists in nature as a saprotroph remains to be determined. Likewise, we have no clear conception of what *Ichthyophonus hoferi* really is, and although it is called a fungus by most researchers working with it, there is little firm evidence to support this viewpoint. There has been a rash of reports recently which describe infections of fishes caused by various Fungi Imperfecti, but we have only vague ideas about how these infections are initiated and no clear ideas at all why particular imperfect fungi cause infections or how one might either prevent or treat these infections if they should ever be the cause of a serious epizootic. What we have tried to do in this book is not only summarize what is known about the fungal diseases of fishes but also to point out some of the areas, both old and new, which are ripe for future mycological investigation.

# OOMYCETES

## MORPHOLOGY AND TAXONOMY

The best known and most widely distributed mycotic infections of fishes are those caused by the freshwater Oomycetes. Indeed, according to Ainsworth (1976), the earliest record of a fungal infection of any vertebrate is that of William Arderon (1748) who illustrated what is obviously an oomycete infection of a roach.

The essential feature which separates the Oomycetes from other classes of fungi is the fact that they produce motile spores with two flagella, one of the whiplash type and the other of the tinsel type, i.e. they are biflagellate heterokont zoospores. The zoospores are produced in structures called zoosporangia and, for most Oomycetes, represent the primary means of asexual reproduction and the primary means of dispersal. Asexual reproduction by means of chlamydospores or gemmae is also common in the Saprolegniales, the order with which this chapter will be most concerned. Sexual reproduction is oogamous and it is from this feature that the class Oomycetes derives its name. Fusion of non-motile gametic nuclei results in the production of a thick-walled resting spore or oospore. Oomycetes also differ from most other fungi in that they have some cellulose in their cell walls and most, if not all, have a diploid nucleus in the vegetative state. Furthermore, all the Oomycetes dealt with in this chapter characteristically have a eucarpic, coenocytic thallus; i.e., they produce filaments called hyphae which, unlike the hyphae of the so-called "higher fungi," have very few septa or cross walls. A mass of hyphae is referred to as a mycelium. Many of these features are illustrated in Figures 1 and 2. A good introduction to the Oomycetes can be found in Webster (1970) and more detailed accounts in Dick (1969, 1973a, b), Sparrow (1973), and Waterhouse (1973a).

The class Oomycetes is divided into four orders: Lagenidiales, Peronosporales, Leptomitales, and Saprolegniales. Species includ-

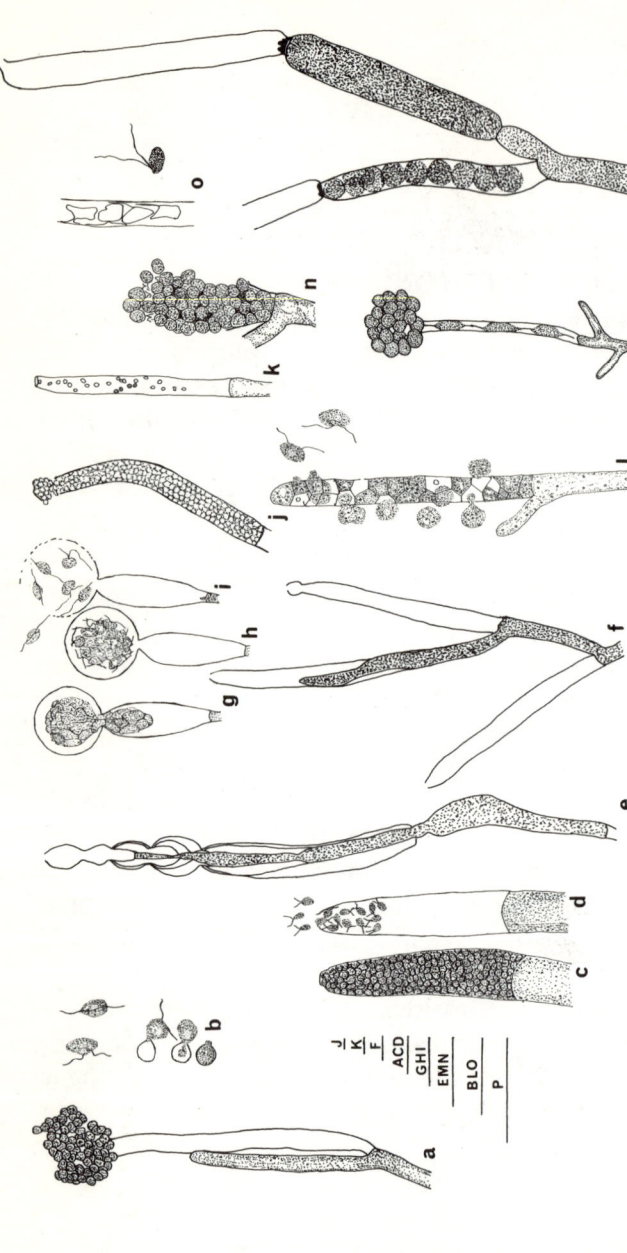

Fig. 1. Zoosporangia of oomycete genera having species potentially parasitic to fish. *a, b*, *Achlya* showing primary cysts clustered around the exit papilla (*a*) and stages in the release of a secondary zoospore from the primary cyst (*b*); *c,d*, *Saprolegnia* showing the mature zoosporangium shortly before (*c*) and during (*d*) release of primary zoospores; *e,f*, examples of internal proliferation, a characteristic means of zoosporangial renewal in *Saprolegnia* species; *g,h,l*, *Pythium* showing stages in the release of zoospores from a vesicle; *i,k*, *Calyptralegnia*; *l*, *Dictyuchus*; *m*, *Aphanomyces*; *n*, *Thraustotheca*; *o*, *Leptolegnia*; *p*, *Leptomitus*. Scale bar = 50 microns. *a-d,l* after Webster (1970); *e,f,o,p* after Coker (1923); *h,n* after Coker & Couch (1924); *g-i* after Goldie-Smith (1952); *m* after Cutter (1941). *Pythiopsis*, recently reported as a parasite of *Perca fluviatilis* by Pickering & Willoughby (1977), has not been included.

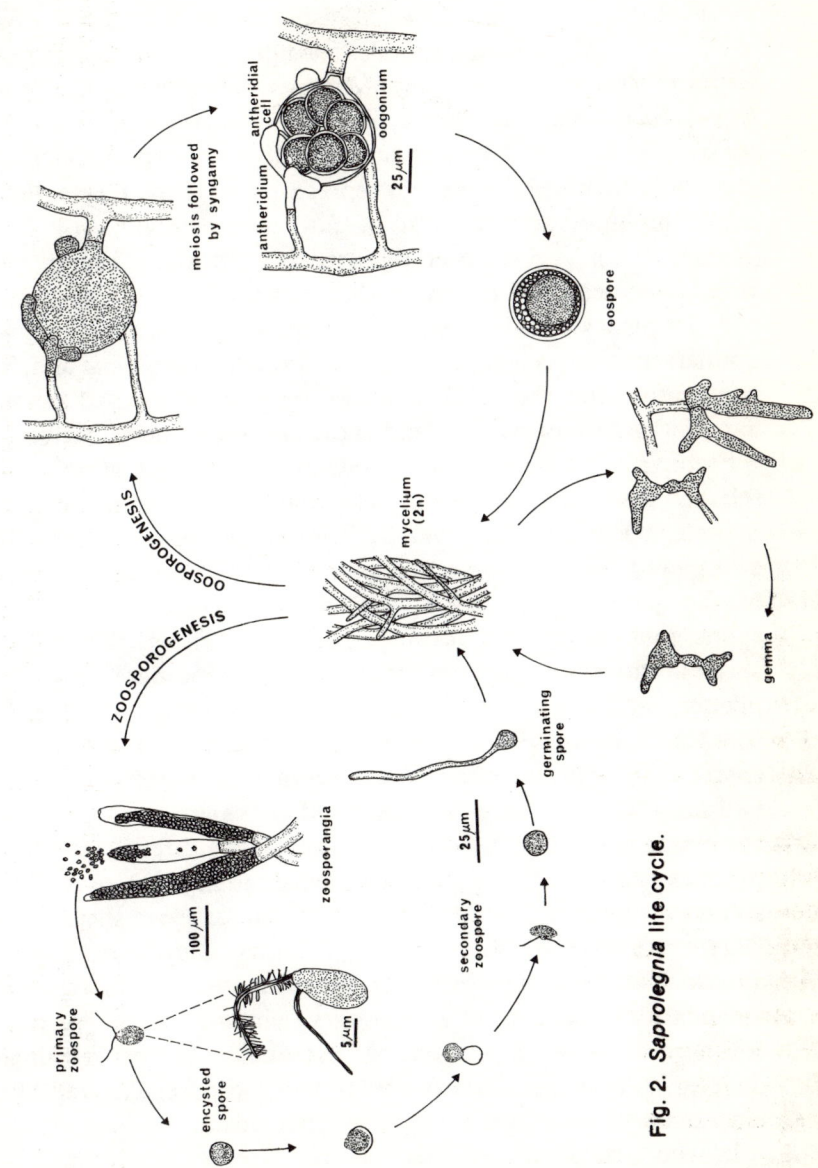

Fig. 2. *Saprolegnia* life cycle.

ed in ten presently recognized oomycete genera have been reported to be either naturally occurring or artificially induced parasites of living fishes (Fig. 1, Table I). Of these, one genus *(Pythium)* is in the Peronosporales, one genus *(Leptomitus)* in the Leptomitales, and eight genera (*Achlya, Aphanomyces, Calyptralegnia, Dictyuchus, Leptolegnia, Pythiopsis, Saprolegnia, Thraustotheca*) are in the Saprolegniales and, more specifically, in the family Saprolegniaceae. No representative of the Lagenidiales [with the dubious exception of *Lagenidium rabenhorstii* Zopf (Kahls, 1930)] has ever been reported as a parasite of fishes. Preeminent among these genera, both in terms of numbers of species and frequency of isolation, are representatives of the two quintessential saprolegnian genera *Achlya* and *Saprolegnia* and, for this reason, the rest of this discussion will be focused on the Saprolegniaceae in general, and these two genera in particular.

Features of zoosporangium production and mode of zoospore release are important for delimiting the genera of the Saprolegniaceae. In the genus *Saprolegnia* the zoospores typically swim away from the zoosporangium prior to encystment whereas in the genus *Achlya* the spores encyst at the mouth of the sporangium where they form a hollow ball (Fig. 1). *Saprolegnia* species characteristically produce two types of zoospores (Fig. 2), a phenomenon referred to as dimorphism. The first or primary zoospore is pip-shaped with the flagella inserted at the tip of the spore. This type of zoospore is generally regarded as a feeble swimmer and it encysts shortly after emergence from the zoosporangium. The cyst may then germinate directly or it may produce another type of zoospore, the secondary zoospore. This secondary zoospore is typically reniform or bean-shaped. Its flagella are inserted laterally with the tinsel flagellum directed anteriorly and the whiplash flagellum directed posteriorly. The secondary zoospore is a much stronger swimmer than the primary zoospore, although it also encysts eventually. It may germinate directly or re-emerge again as a secondary zoospore. This repeated emergence of zoospores is called polyplanetism.

In the genus *Achlya* there is no free-swimming primary zoospore. Secondary zoospores emerge from the cysts at the mouth of the sporangium. In *Aphanomyces* encystment also occurs at the mouth of the zoosporangium in a manner similar to *Achlya*.

# TABLE I

## Species of Oomycetes reported as parasites of fishes.[1]

| Fungi | References |
|---|---|
| **SAPROLEGNIALES** | |
| **Saprolegniaceae** | |
| *Achlya* spp. | Tiffney, 1939a; Vishniac & Nigrelli, 1957; Willoughby, 1970; Bhargava, Swarup & Singh, 1971; Nolard-Tintigner, 1973, 1974; Srivastava, 1976; Pickering & Willoughby, 1977; Jha, Seth & Srivastava, 1977 |
| *Achlya ambisexualis* Raper | Vishniac & Nigrelli, 1957; Willoughby, 1970; Nolard-Tintigner, 1973, 1974 |
| *Achlya americana* Humphrey[2] | Scott & Warren, 1964 |
| *Achlya bisexualis* Coker & Couch | Vishniac & Nigrelli, 1957; O'Bier, 1960; Scott & O'Bier, 1962 |
| *Achlya caroliniana* Coker[3] | Srivastava, 1976; Srivastava & Srivastava, 1977 |
| *Achlya diffusa* Harvey ex Johnson[3] | Srivastava, 1976 |
| *Achlya dubia* Coker | Bhargava, Swarup & Singh, 1971; Srivastava, 1976 |
| *Achlya flagellata* Coker | Tiffney & Wolf, 1937; Tiffney, 1939a; Domashova, 1971; Srivastava, 1976 |
| *Achlya intricata* Beneke | Howard, Seymour & Johnson, 1970 |
| *Achlya klebsiana* Pieters[2] | Vishniac & Nigrelli, 1957 |
| *Achlya orion* Coker & Couch | Srivastava, 1976 |

[1]This list does not include species isolated only from dead fishes or fish eggs but does include most, if not all, species reported as naturally occurring or experimentally induced parasites of fishes.
[2]Species reported only as experimentally induced parasites and not as naturally occurring isolates.
[3]Species reported as experimentally induced parasites which may also be naturally occurring parasites. The reports of Srivastava (1976) for *Achlya caroliniana, A. diffusa, A. proliferoides, Aphanomyces laevis* and *Dichtyuchus sterile* and of Scott & Warren (1964) and Stuart & Fuller (1968) for *Pythium* spp. are unclear on this point.

| Fungi | References |
|---|---|
| *Achlya prolifera* Nees von Esenbeck[4] | Nolard-Tintigner, 1974; Srivastava, 1976; Srivastava & Srivastava, 1977a |
| *Achlya proliferoides* Coker[3] | Srivastava, 1976 |
| *Achlya racemosa* Hildebrand[2] | Hoshina, Sano & Sunayama, 1960 |
| *Achlya sparrovii* Reischer[2] (= *A. racemosa*, Johnson, 1956) | Vishniac & Nigrelli, 1957 |
| *Aphanomyces* spp. | Shanor & Saslow, 1944; Willoughby, 1970; Srivastava, 1976; Pickering & Willoughby, 1977 |
| *Aphanomyces laevis* de Bary[3] | Vishniac & Nigrelli, 1957; Srivastava, 1976 |
| *Aphanomyces stellatus* de Bary[2] | Hoshina, Sano & Sunayama, 1960 |
| *Calyptralegnia achlyoides* (Coker & Couch) Coker[2] | Vishniac & Nigrelli, 1957 |
| *Dictyuchus* sp.[2] | Nolard-Tintigner, 1974; Tiffney, 1939a |
| *Dictyuchus anomalus* Nagai | Srivastava, 1976; Srivastava & Srivastava, 1977b |
| *Dictyuchus monosporus* Leitgeb[2] | Nolard-Tintigner, 1974 |
| *Dictyuchus sterile* Coker[3] | Srivastava, 1976 |
| *Isoachlya anisospora* var. *indica* Saksena & Bhargava[2] ( = *Saprolegnia diclina*, Seymour, 1970) | Srivastava, 1976 |
| *Isoachlya monilifera* de Bary[2] (= *Saprolegnia unispora*, Seymour, 1970) | Vishniac & Nigrelli, 1957 |

[4]These are recent references to infection of fishes by this species. *A. prolifera* was commonly reported as a parasite of fishes by earlier authors but these references have not been included because we are either not sure that the isolate was obtained from a living fish or not sure that the isolate was properly identified.

*Isoachlya unispora* Coker & Couch
(= *Saprolegnia unispora*, Seymour, 1970)   Domashova, 1971

*Leptolegnia caudata* de Bary
*Protoachlya paradoxa* Coker[2]
(= *Achlya* (-proto) *paradoxa*, Dick, 1973a)   Willoughby, 1970
Vishniac & Nigrelli, 1957

*Pythiopsis* sp.
*Saprolegnia* spp. (Also includes non-fruiting isolates classified as *Saprolegnia parasitica* Coker or one of its synonyms as cited by Seymour, 1970.)   Pickering & Willoughby, 1977
Huxley, 1882a, b; Clinton, 1894; Johnston, 1917; Coker, 1923; Duff, 1930; Tiffney, 1939a, b; Chidambaram, 1942; Chaudhuri, Kochhar, Lotus, Banjeree & Khan, 1947; Aleem, Ruivo & Théodoridès, 1953; Lennon, 1954; Vishniac & Nigrelli, 1957; Arasaki, Nozawa & Miyake, 1958; O'Bier, 1960; Scott & O'Bier, 1962; Scott & Warren, 1964; Dudka, 1964; Stuart & Fuller, 1968; Bhargava, Swarup & Singh, 1971; Nolard-Tintigner, 1971, 1973; Bootsma, 1973; Johnson, 1974; Srivastava, 1976; Neish, 1976, 1977; Hatai, Eugusa & Nomura, 1977; Pickering & Willoughby, 1977 Hatai, Egusa & Nomura, 1977; Pickering & Willoughby, 1977

*Saprolegnia australis* Elliot
*Saprolegnia delica* Coker
(= *S. diclina*, Seymour, 1970)
*Saprolegnia diclina* Humphrey   Vishniac & Nigrelli, 1957; O'Bier, 1960; Scott & O'Bier, 1962; Dudka & Florinskaya, 1971; Nolard-Tintigner, 1973
McKay, 1967; Willoughby, 1970; Nolard-Tintigner, 1970, 1973; Srivastava, 1976; Miyazaki, Kubota & Tashiro, 1977; Hatai & Egusa, 1977

*Saprolegnia diclina* Humphrey Type I
*Saprolegnia ferax* (Gruithuisen) Thuret   Willoughby, 1968, 1969, 1971, 1972, 1978

Tiffney, 1939a; Vishniac & Nigrelli, 1957; O'Bier, 1960; Hoshina, Sano & Sunayama, 1960; Scott & O'Bier, 1962; Nolard-Tintigner, 1970, 1971, 1973; Bhargava, Swarup & Singh, 1971; Srivastava, 1976; Srivastava & Srivastava, 1977c

| | |
|---|---|
| *Saprolegnia invaderis* Davis & Lazar (= *S. ferax*, Seymour, 1970) | Davis & Lazar, 1941 |
| *Saprolegnia megasperma* Coker[2] (=*S. ferax*, Seymour, 1970) | Vishniac & Nigrelli, 1957 |
| *Saprolegnia mixta* de Bary | Vishniac & Nigrelli, 1957; Dudka & Florinskaya, 1971 |
| *Saprolegnia monoica* Pringsheim (= *S. ferax*, Seymour, 1970) | O'Bier, 1960; Scott & O'Bier, 1962; Domashova, 1971 |
| *Saprolegnia parasitica* Coker emend. Kanouse | Rucker, 1944; Hoshina, Sano & Sunayama, 1960; O'Bier, 1960; Scott & O'Bier, 1962; Nolard-Tintigner, 1973; Srivastava, 1976 |
| *Saprolegnia shikotsuensis* Hatai, Egusa & Awakura | Hatai, Egusa & Awakura, 1977 |
| *Saprolegnia subterranea* (Dissmann) Seymour | Pickering & Willoughby, 1977 |
| *Thraustotheca clavata* (de Bary) Humphrey[2] | Vishniac & Nigrelli, 1957 |
| *Thraustotheca primoachlya* Coker & Couch[2] (Dick, 1973a, suggested that this species should be placed in the genus *Achlya*.) | Vishniac & Nigrelli, 1957 |

## LEPTOMITALES
### Leptomitaceae
*Leptomitus lacteus* (Roth) Agardh — Lennon, 1954; Willoughby, 1970; Pickering & Willoughby, 1977

## PERONOSPORALES
### Pythiaceae
*Pythium* sp.[3] — Scott & Warren, 1964

*Aphanomyces* is distinguished from *Achlya* by its more delicate hyphae and by the fact that its zoospores typically occur in a single row in the zoosporangium. In the genus *Dictyuchus,* encystment occurs within the zoosporangium and secondary zoospores emerge independently through separate pores.

Although variations in zoospore release are used for delimiting saprolegnian genera, it must be noted that these mechanisms are subject to environmental and nutritional modification. For example, Salvin (1941) and Scott (1956) have shown that temperature can have an effect on zoospore motility, causing a *Saprolegnia* isolate to behave like an *Achlya* or an *Aphanomyces* isolate to behave like a *Leptolegnia*. With reference to nutrients, it has been shown that a deficiency of calcium ions can affect zoosporogenesis in *Achlya* (Griffin, 1966). *Saprolegnia* species growing on fish frequently exhibit aplanetism (Neish, 1977). In this case zoospores encyst and germinate within the zoosporangium and the germ tubes penetrate the sporangial wall (Fig. 3). This phenomenon is frequently associated with "staling" of cultures and with bacterial

Fig. 3. Aplanoid zoosporangium showing *in situ* germination of zoospores. Scale bar = 50 microns. (From Journal of Fish Biology, Academic Press, Inc. (London) Ltd.)

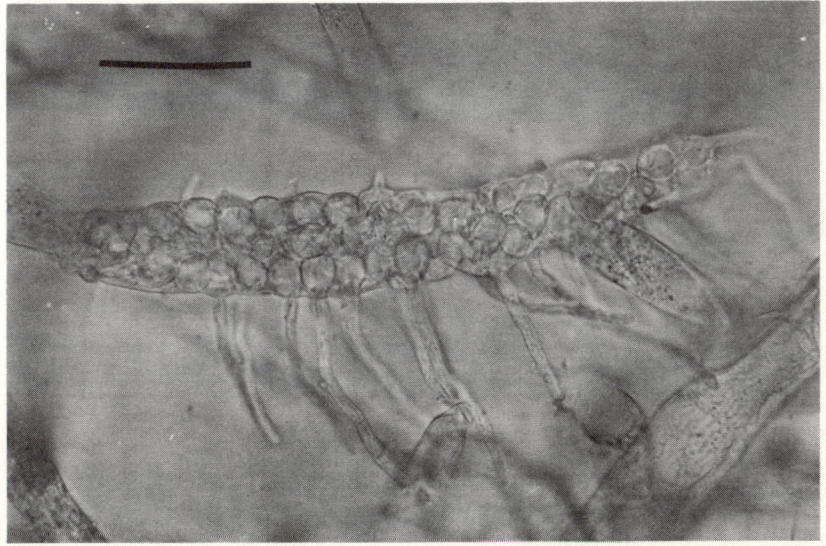

contamination but, apart from these observations, little work has been done to elucidate the mechanisms which lead to this condition. Another question is the degree to which zoosporangial characteristics, even under "normal" conditions, can be used to resolve genera with respect to their degree of genetic relatedness. For example, recent DNA base composition work, while hardly conclusive, suggests that the genus *Saprolegnia* is composed of much more homogeneous elements than the genus *Achlya* (Green & Dick, 1972; Neish & Green, 1976).

While characteristics of zoosporangium formation and zoospore release are important for delimitation of saprolegnian genera, morphological variations of the sexual reproductive structures are important for delimiting taxa within genera. Saprolegnian fungi produce morphologically distinct gametangia. The male gametangium is called an antheridium and the female gametangium, an oogonium (Fig. 2). Some species, notably many isolates of *Saprolegnia ferax,* do not produce antheridia and the oospores develop parthenogenetically. A few species in the genera *Achlya* and *Dictyuchus* are heterothallic and reproduce sexually only when opposite mating strains are brought together, the one strain bearing antheridia and the other strain oogonia. In most species, however, cultures derived from a single uninucleate spore will give rise to a mycelium which typically bears both antheridia and oogonia; i.e., they are homothallic. In these cases, the origin of the antheridial branch can be an important diagnostic criterion. If the antheridial cell is borne on the oogonial stalk directly beneath the oogonium it is called an hypogynous antheridial cell. If the antheridial branch comes from the oogonial stalk it is an androgynous antheridium. If it comes from the same hypha as the oogonium, but does not come from the oogonial stalk, it is a monoclinous antheridium and if the antheridial branch comes from another hypha, it is a diclinous antheridium as illustrated in Figure 2.

Meiosis occurs in both the antheridial cell and the oogonium and, since discrete male gametes are never formed, there has to be gametangial contact to effect fertilization. This process has been reviewed recently by Beakes & Gay (1977). Following fertilization, oospheres in the oogonium become oospores and the evidence for this is the development of a thick wall and a distinct redistribution of the protoplasmic contents. In the Saprolegniaceae, the oospore has a central ooplast (Howard, 1971) with a somewhat granular appearance and a large amount of lipidlike material which probably represents a food reserve. This material may occur as a single eccentric globule or it may consist of many globules dispersed around the ooplast. If the ooplast is displaced slightly to one side, as shown in Figure 2, it is called a subcentric oospore. Saprolegnian oospores are notoriously reluctant to germinate. This aspect of their biology has been discussed by Dick (1972) and Dick & Win—Tin (1973). When an oospore does germinate, it produces a hypha which may or may not be terminated by a zoosporangium.

## INVESTIGATIONS OF SAPROLEGNIOSIS: A BRIEF HISTORICAL OUTLINE

Since Oomycetes that infect fishes produce an easily recognized cottony mycelium on the surface of the affected animal .(Plates 1-4), they have probably been recognized since antiquity. Published reports from Europe describing these infections date from the mid-eighteenth century (Arderon, 1748; Spallanzani, 1777, cited by Ramsbottom, 1916; Shrank, 1789, cited by Humphrey, 1893) and, for the next century, interested observers continued to discuss the identity of these fungi and their effect on freshwater animals (Hannover, 1839, 1842, cited by Buchwald, 1971; Bennet, 1842; Goodsir, 1842; Areshoug, 1844; Unger, 1844; Robin, 1853; Berkeley, 1864).

In 1877 Oomycetes were reported for the first time in the European literature in association with an epizootic which came to be called the "salmon disease." This disease was first observed in rivers near the border between England and Scotland but later spread to other rivers in Great Britain and became a source of great concern. An inquiry was set up and the results were presented to both Houses of Parliament in 1880 (Buckland, Walpole & Young, 1880). The Commissioners of the inquiry were unable to reach any conclusions about the causes, spread, or treatment of the disease and prophetically suggested that ". . . increased observations by naturalists, microscopists, and other scientific persons, prolonged over many seasons, may possibly be necessary in order to enable us to arrive at a complete knowledge of the cause of the recent outbreak of *Saprolegnia*, and the remedies which are applicable to this disease."

Some observers felt that the "salmon disease" was caused by the fungus (Stirling, 1879-80; Huxley, 1882a, b), whereas others felt that the fungus was the mere consequence of a disease brought on by various predisposing factors. There was a diversity of opinion as to what these predisposing factors might be and the list included pollution, low water levels, overcrowding of fish, obstruction by weirs, failure to remove dead fish from the water, and wounding of fish caused by fighting on the spawning beds or by anglers.

It was popularly assumed that the fungus associated with the 1877-1881 epizootic of British salmon was *Saprolegnia ferax* and the terms *Saprolegnia* and *Saprolegnia ferax* often seem to have been used interchangeably. The literature of the era, however, provides no clear evidence that the fungus growing on the fish was actually *S. ferax*. This has been documented by Neish (1976) who concurred with earlier opinions expressed by Edington (1899) and Coker (1923) who noted that the fungi infecting fish were ". . . for a long time carelessly spoken of as *S. ferax*." We can now be quite certain that the fungus associated with the "salmon disease" was definitely not *S. ferax*. The "salmon disease" of 1877-1881 is now regarded, on the basis of clinical evidence, as the first well documented epizootic attributed to the disease now known as Ulcerative Dermal Necrosis (UDN) of salmonids (Roberts, 1972; Murphy, 1973). Extensive investigations of the fungal component of UDN have shown it to be a particular strain of *Saprolegnia* which is now designated as *Saprolegnia diclina* Type I (Willoughby, 1969, 1971, 1977, 1978). Moreover, *Saprolegnia diclina* Type I appears to be similar in many respects to the *Saprolegnia* sp. Category D isolates described by Neish (1977) as parasites of Pacific salmon (*Oncorhynchus* spp.) in British Columbia. This suggests that there may be a particular strain of *Saprolegnia* with a proclivity toward being a parasite of salmonid fish.

Most early investigations of the "salmon disease" did not consider that organisms other than *Saprolegnia* might be associated with the disease. The science of bacteriology was in its infancy and viruses were unknown, situations which, along with the fact that the fungus was such an obvious component of the disease, probably account for this lack of interest. In view of this, it is interesting to note that as early as 1880, Rutherford suggested that bacteria might be an important component of the "salmon disease" (Rutherford, 1881). M.C. Cooke, a leading mycologist of the day, scoffed at Rutherford's suggestion (Cooke, 1880), but in 1903 Rutherford was apparently vindicated by J. Hume Patterson whose carefully executed study of the "salmon disease" seemed to demonstrate conclusively that the disease was caused by a motile, gram-negative bacillus that Hume Patterson named *Bacillus Salmonis Pestis*. Hume Patterson's study, in an historical sense, marks the end of the investigations initiated by the 1877 epizootic and was, for many years, generally accepted as the solution to the problem of the cause of the "salmon disease" (Drew, 1909; Smith, 1912; Rushton, 1925).

The late nineteenth and early twentieth century was an era of considerable taxonomic development for the Saprolegniaceae and, because taxonomic concepts had not stabilized, an era of considerable taxonomic and nomenclatural confusion. Fungi isolated from fish and fish eggs were no exception to this rule and during this period a number of species were described, or isolates named, which have subsequently been set aside as excluded or doubtful taxa, or have been reduced to synonymy in recent monographs. These are shown in Table II. In addition, problems centering around the careless use of the name *Saprolegnia ferax* were compounded by the fact that there was an overlapping equivocal use of the name *Achlya prolifera*. *A. prolifera* was described originally by C.G. Nees von Esenbeck in 1823 (see discussion in Johnson, 1956), but later, in 1851, Pringsheim applied the same name to an isolate which is now considered to be *Saprolegnia ferax* (Seymour, 1970). Hence, there is the dual problem that some organisms referred to as *S. ferax* may not have been that species (and, in the case of the "salmon disease fungus," almost certainly were not that species) whereas other isolates, referred to as *A. prolifera*, may indeed have been *S. ferax*.

The late nineteenth and early twentieth century was also an era of rapid development of aquaculture facilities in Europe and North America, and it soon became apparent to workers in Austria (Fiessiger, 1903), Canada (Harrison, 1918; Huntsman, 1918), France (Valery-Mayet, 1885; Vincent, 1908; Griffon & Maublanc,

## TABLE II

Nomenclatural status of some isolates of *Achlya* and *Saprolegnia* obtained from fishes or fish eggs prior to 1923.

| Species | Isolated from | Reference | Present Status |
|---|---|---|---|
| *Achlya hoferi* Harz | mirror carp | Harz, 1906 | A taxon of doubtful affinities (Johnson, 1956). Also see discussion of *A. treleaseana* by Howard, Seymour & Johnson (1970). |
| *Achlya nowickii* Raciborski | carp | Raciborski, 1886 | Excluded taxon (Johnson, 1956). Also see discussion of *A. treleaseana* by Howard, Seymour & Johnson (1970). |
| *Achlya prolifera* C.G. Nees | goldfish, Japanese fighting fish, *Oryzias latipes*, Gusai-chi | Sawada, 1912, 1919 (cited by Wolf, 1939) | May be *Achlya flagellata* Coker (Johnson, 1956). |
| *Achlya racemosa* var. *stelligera* Cornu | trout eggs | Humphrey, 1893 | Synonymn of *Achlya colorata* Pringsheim (Johnson, 1956). |
| *Achlya radiosa* Maurizio | eggs of American brook trout living pike | Maurizio, 1899 | Still thought to be a valid species (Johnson, 1956). |
| *Saprolegnia esocina* Maurizio | | Maurizio, 1896 | Synonym of *Saprolegnia ferax* (Gruith.) Thuret (Seymour, 1970). |
| *Saprolegnia floccosa* Maurizio | eggs of American brook trout | Maurizio, 1899 | Synonym of *S. ferax* (Seymour, 1970). |
| *Saprolegnia paradoxa* Maurizio | eggs of sea trout | Maurizio, 1899 | Synonym of *S. ferax* (Seymour, 1970). |
| *Saprolegnia hypogyna* var. *Coregoni* Maurizio | *Coregonus* sp. egg | Maurizio, 1899 | Synonym of *Saprolegnia hypogyna* (Pringsheim) de Bary (Seymour, 1970). |

1911), Germany (Benecke, 1886; Maurizio, 1895, 1896, 1897a, b, 1899), Poland (Walentowicz, 1885; Raciborski, 1886), and the United States (Ryder, 1881, 1883; Humphrey, 1893; Henshall, 1898) that saprolegnian fungi posed a threat to a variety of freshwater fishes at all phases of their life cycle. The observations of these workers were augmented by others who described infections in aquaria (Clark, 1874; Clinton, 1894) and natural waters (Schnetzler, 1887; Blanc, 1888; Hardy, 1910; Johnston, 1917).

W.C. Coker's classical monograph, *The Saprolegniaceae with notes on other water molds*, appeared in 1923. It was in this volume that Coker described *Saprolegnia parasitica,* defying a venerable taxonomic tradition in the process by ignoring the necessity of observing oogonia before the isolate could be described or identified. Coker essentially defined *S. parasitica* on the basis of the substratum (fishes or fish eggs) from which it was obtained, and the fact that it did not produce oogonia under normal culture conditions. Thus, when Kanouse (1932) isolated some *Saprolegnia* spp. from fishes and fish eggs, she assumed they were, *ipso facto, S. parasitica.* Kanouse found oogonia in some of her cultures, noted that they were distinct from the oogonia of fungi belonging to the *S. ferax* group, and went on to describe *S. parasitica* as a morphologically and physiologically distinct entity without ever noting the obvious similarity of her isolates to *Saprolegnia diclina.* Kanouse (1932) also reported several nutritional experiments which apparently convinced both Coker (Coker & Mathews, 1937) and Tiffney (1939a) that *S. parasitica* would not produce oogonia except when it was grown on special media. This is not true. It is quite clear that Kanouse observed oogonia in cultures grown on hemp seeds in distilled water (a routine procedure nowadays). In fact, Kanouse's description of *S. parasitica* was based predominantly on its appearance in the hemp seed cultures which she said ". . . in many respects. . . appear more normal."

The main diagnostic features of *S. parasitica* Coker emend. Kanouse when grown on hemp seeds were its thin, unpitted oogonial walls, diclinous antheridia, and small (18-22 microns), subcentric (sensu Coker, 1923) oospores. Coker (Coker & Mathews, 1937) incorporated Kanouse's description into his later description of *S. parasitica;* therefore, it may be assumed that he accepted Kanouse's emended description even though it was not based on his type material.

Hence, the modern concept of *Saprolegnia parasitica* dates from 1932, or at least from no later than 1937, and after this date the authors should not have used this name for isolates that did not produce oogonia. Unfortunately, this did not happen and numerous authors (e.g., Tiffney, 1939a, b; Sparrow, 1952; Burrows, 1949; Hoshina & Ookubo, 1956; Dayal, 1958; Wolf, 1958; Schmitt & Beneke, 1962; Lee, 1962; Gopalakrishnan, 1965, 1968; Bhargava, Swarup & Singh, 1971; Cline & Post, 1972; Volz & Beneke, 1972; Johnson, 1974) continued to use the name *S. parasitica* in its original sense or at least without making it clear that it was not used in its original sense.

O'Bier (1960) was among the first to emphasize the undesirability of this practice. He wrote:

"The use of asexual characters and the parasitic habit as the diagnostic features for this species have made the taxon the 'catch-all' for all non-fruiting isolates of *Saprolegnia* even though reproductive structures have been described for the species. . . .

"The author believes that the easiest and least hazardous solution to this problem for the present is to include in *S. parasticia* only those fungi that have exhibited sexuality and possess the diagnostic features of the taxon."

The name *Saprolegnia parasitica* then, can be, and clearly has been, used in two different senses. First, the name can be used as a convenient repository for any *Saprolegnia* isolate which appears unable to produce oogonia and has been obtained from fishes or fish eggs. Furthermore, this identification can be made without making any serious attempt to culture these organisms under conditions that might encourage oogonium formation even though it has been clearly established that environmental factors such as temperature and light can affect oogonium formation in *Saprolegnia* isolates (Krause, 1960; Szaniszlo, 1965; Lee & Scott, 1967; Neish, 1975a, 1977). On the other hand, the name *Saprolegnia parasitica* can also refer to those *Saprolegnia* isolates with thin oogonial walls, predominantly diclinous antheridia, and subcentric oospores, regardless of the source of the isolates.

The use of the name *Saprolegnia parasitica* in these different senses has led to confusion and inaccuracy. It has, in many cases, provided a facile solution to what is, in reality, a difficult taxonomic problem. It has also, occasionally, lent an aura of false respectability to poorly studied, and possibly incorrectly identified, *Saprolegnia* isolates. As a partial solution to this problem, Neish (1976) proposed that the name *Saprolegnia parasitica* should be rejected as a nomen ambiguum in accordance with Article 69 of the International Code of Botanical Nomenclature (Stafleu et al., 1972). Neish (1976) argued that characteristics such as mean oospore size and oospore type (centric or subcentric)—characters previously thought to have great value for separating *S. parasitica* from the other *Saprolegnia* species with predominantly diclinous antheridia—were of little diagnostic value. Given acceptance of these assumptions, Neish noted that all fruiting isolates of *S. parasitica* could be correctly assigned to *Saprolegnia diclina* Humphrey without violating Humphrey's (1893) concept of this species. This view has not yet been formally proposed in the mycological literature but there has been a tendency recently for mycologists working with these fungi to refer them to the *S. diclina-S. parasitica* complex. This complex, besides including *S. diclina* and *S. parasitica*, also includes *S. kauffmaniana* Pieters, Willoughby's *Saprolegnia* sp. Type 1 (now called *S. diclina* Type 1), the *Saprolegnia* isolates described by Neish (1976, 1977) and the recently described *S. shikotsuensis* Hatai, Egusa & Awakura (1977). *Saprolegnia australis* Elliot arguably belongs to this group as well. Records of these fungi as fish parasites are given in Table I.

Willoughby (1978) recently discussed the taxonomy of the *S. diclina-S. parasitica* complex in some detail. He has adopted the suggestion by Neish (1976) that *S. parasitica* Coker emend. Kanouse be considered a synonym of *S. diclina* and, on the basis of his work with these fungi in the English Lake District, has divided *S. diclina* into three subspecific groups, basing the separation on growth characteristics with special emphasis on the length/breadth ratio of the oogonium. He noted that only his *S. diclina* Type 1 occurs as a parasite on salmonid fish, that only his *S. diclina* Type 2 occurs as a parasite on perch *(Perca fluviatilis* L.), and that *S. diclina* Type 3 was purely saprotrophic.

Besides Kanouse's (1932) paper on *S. parasitica*, there were several other significant papers concerning saprolegniosis published in the nineteen-thirties including a major review in Russian by Shereshevskaya (1932), a study of the water mould population of a fish hatchery by Monsma (1937), and a study of the taxonomy and pathology of the fungi causing saprolegniosis in the northeastern United States (Tiffney, 1939a, b).

In 1941, Davis & Lazar described *Saprolegnia invaderis (= S. ferax)* which they reported as the cause of an alimentary tract infection of rainbow trout *(Salmo gairdneri)* fingerlings. This report and Agersborg's (1933) report of "intestinal fungisitosis" of brook trout *(Salvelinus fontinalis)* fingerlings were the only ones describing the initial site of a saprolegnian infection as the gut instead of a site somewhere on the surface of the fish (e.g., skin, gills, nares) until recently, when this phenomenon was confirmed by Miyazaki, Kubota & Tashiro (1977) and by Hatai & Egusa (1977). These workers found that *Saprolegnia diclina* infected the guts of rainbow trout and amago salmon *(Oncorhynchus rhodurus* f. *macrostomus)* fry, sometimes in association with an as yet unidentified filamentous fungus with septate hyphae. Saprolegnian fungi are not restricted to living as parasites of the skin, gills, and musculature (Bootsma, 1973; Nolard-Tintigner, 1973, 1974); nonetheless, reports of these infections being initiated in the gut are remarkable.

Rucker (1944) carried out the first detailed study of saprolegniosis of Pacific salmon *(Oncorhynchus* spp.). He concluded that the fungus, which he identified as *Saprolegnia parasitica* Coker sensu Kanouse, was a secondary invader which could not normally initiate an infection and that the primary cause of the infections was the myxobacterium *Flexibacter columnaris*. Subsequent studies of saprolegniosis of Pacific salmon (McKay, 1967; Neish, 1976), while not refuting Rucker's observations, have strongly promoted the viewpoint that saprolegnian fungi can cause primary infections of Pacific salmon. This apparent discrepancy will be discussed in the next section of this chapter.

Two notable studies carried out in the nineteen-fifties are those by Lennon (1954) and by Vishniac & Nigrelli (1957). Lennon found that *Leptomitus lacteus* was associated with wounds of fish caused by sea lampreys *(Petromyzon marinus)*. This is one of the few reports (Table I) which record *L. lacteus* as a parasite of living fishes. Vishniac & Nigrelli (1957) used a variety of fungi (Table I) to infect a single species of fish *(Xiphophorus maculatus)*. Their study complements that of Tiffney (1939b) who used a single fungal isolate to infect a variety of fishes (Table III).

In 1964, an epizootic of Atlantic salmon *(Salmo salar)* was noted in southern Eire and subsequently spread to Great Britain (Munro, 1970) and continental Europe (de Kinkelin & Turdu, 1971). At the present time the disease appears to have waned, but from 1966-1974 it was a source of considerable concern and, consequently, the subject of much research and numerous review articles (Pyefinch & Elson, 1967; Elson, 1968; Carbery, 1968; Carbery & Strickland, 1968; Strickland & Carbery, 1968; Munro, 1970; Stevenson, 1970; Roberts, 1972; Murphy, 1973; Wilson, 1976).

The detailed clinical descriptions by Huxley (1882a, b), Edington (1889), and others noted previously, leave little reason to doubt that this latest epizootic was virtually identical to the 1877 epizootic and the disease is now universally referred to as Ulcerative Dermal Necrosis (UDN) (Roberts, 1972). UDN is considered to be a disease which is distinct from the "normal" saprolegniosis associated with debilitated or sexually mature fish (Roberts & Shepherd, 1974; Bauduoy & Tuffery, 1973).

A key feature of UDN is lesions which occur on the non-scaled areas of the body, especially the head. The first lesions are small, oval, blanched patches which frequently become ulcerated and then hemorrhagic (Fig. 4). The cause of these intial lesions is unknown. A favored hypothesis is that they are caused by an epitheliotropic virus (Roberts, 1972; O'Brien, 1974), but as yet there is no direct evidence to support this hypothesis (Hill, 1976; Meier, Klinger & Mueller, 1977; Meier, Klinger, Mueller & Luginbuehl, 1977). Whether or not a virus is involved, it appears that stress (O'Brien, 1974; Reichenbach-Klinke, 1974) and possibly the presence of sublethal concentrations of pollutants (Reichenbach-Klinke, 1975; Wachs, 1973) may also contribute to the development of the disease. Parenthetically, it should be noted that since sublethal concentrations of pollutants can involve a stress response (Donaldson & Dye, 1975), these two factors cannot be considered as unrelated. Meier, Klinger & Mueller (1977) recently

## TABLE III

**Species of teleost fishes successfully infected experimentally by saprolegnian fungi.**

| Species | References |
|---|---|
| ANABANTIDAE | |
| *Anabas testudineus* (Bloch) | Srivastava & Srivastava, 1977a |
| *Colisa fasciata* (Bloch & Schneider) | Srivastava, 1976; Srivastava & Srivastava, 1977a, c |
| *Colisa lalia* (Hamilton-Buchanan) | Srivastava, 1976; Srivastava & Srivastava, 1977a, b |
| *Helostoma temmincki* Cuvier & Valenciennes | Scott & Warren, 1964 |
| ANGUILLIDAE | |
| *Anguilla japonica* Temminck & Schlegel | Hoshina & Ookubo, 1956; Hoshina, Sano & Sunayama, 1960 |
| CATOSTOMIDAE | |
| *Erimyzon sucetta* (Lacépède) | Tiffney, 1939b |
| CENTRARCHIDAE | |
| *Lepomis gibbosus* (Linnaeus) (cited as *Eupomius gibbosus*) | Tiffney, 1939b |
| *Micropterus salmoides* (Lacépède) | Tiffney, 1939b |
| *Pomoxis nigromaculatus* (Lesueur) (cited as *P. sparoides*) | Tiffney, 1939b |
| CICHLIDAE | |
| *Tilapia* sp | Nolard-Tintigner, 1970 |
| CYPRINIDAE | |
| *Carassius auratus* (Linnaeus) | Tiffney, 1939b |
| *Cirrhinus mrigala* (Hamilton-Buchanan) | Srivastava & Srivastava, 1977c |
| *Puntius sophore* (Hamilton-Buchanan) | Srivastava, 1976; Srivastava & Srivastava, 1977a, b, c |
| *Semotilus atromaculatus* (Mitchill) | Tiffney, 1939b |

| Species | References |
|---|---|
| **CYPRINODONTIDAE** | |
| *Fundulus heteroclitus* (Linnaeus) | Tiffney & Wolf, 1937; Tiffney, 1939b |
| *Poecilia reticulata* Peters (cited as *Lebistes reticulatus*) | Tiffney, 1939b; Scott & Warren, 1964; Nolard-Tintigner, 1970, 1971, 1973, 1974 |
| *Mollienesia latipinna* Lesueur | Scott & Warren, 1964 |
| *Xiphophorus helleri* Heckel | Scott & Warren, 1964; Nolard-Tintigner, 1970, 1971, 1973, 1974 |
| *Xiphophorus maculatus* (Guenther) | Vishniac & Nigrelli, 1957; Scott & Warren, 1964 |
| **ESOCIDAE** | |
| *Esox niger* Lesueur (cited as *E. reticulatus*) | Tiffney, 1939b |
| **ICTALURIDAE** | |
| *Ictalurus nebulosus* Lesueur (cited as *Ameiurus nebulosus*) | Tiffney, 1939b |
| **NETOPTERIDAE** | |
| *Notopterus chitala* (Hamilton-Buchanan) | Srivastava & Srivastava, 1977a |
| **PERCICHTHYIDAE** | |
| *Morone americana* (Gmelin) | Tiffney, 1939b |
| **PERCIDAE** | |
| *Perca flavescens* (Mitchill) | Tiffney, 1939b |
| **SALMONIDAE** | |
| *Oncorhynchus kisutch* (Walbaum) | McKay, 1967; Neish, 1976 |
| *Salmo gairdneri* Richardson (cited as *S. irideus*) | Tiffney, 1939b |
| *Salmo salar* Linnaeus (cited as *S. sebago*) | Tiffney, 1939b |
| *Salmo trutta* Linnaeus (cited as *S. fario*) | Tiffney, 1939b |

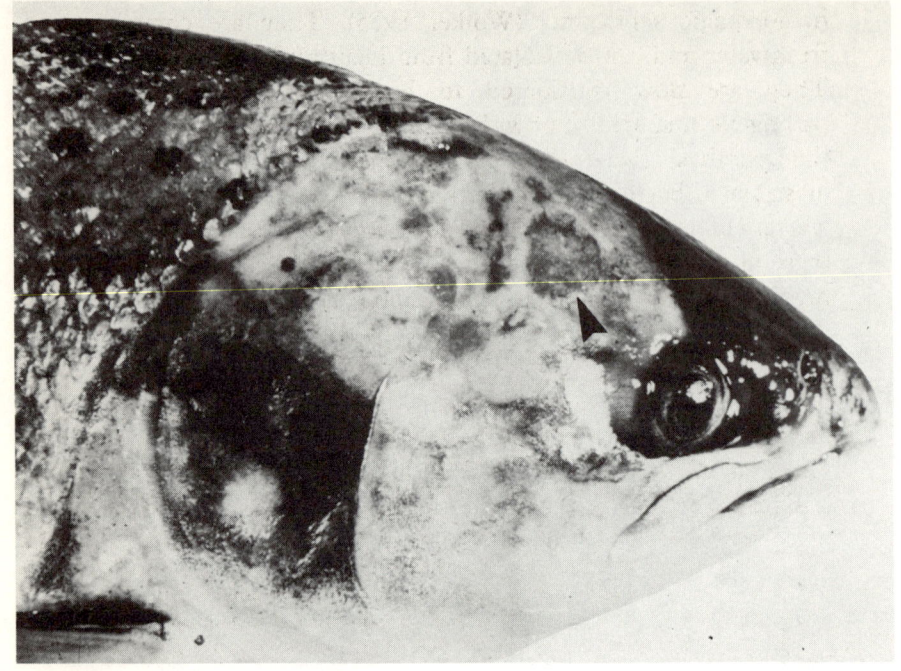

Fig. 4. Head of a salmon (*Salmo salar*) suffering from ulcerative dermal necrosis (UDN) showing both complete ulcertation (arrow) and less severe lesions. (Photograph courtesy of R. J. Roberts, W. M. Shearer, A. L. S. Munro, and K. G. R. Elson, with permission of the Journal of Pathology.)

presented a detailed discussion of the etiology of UDN.

The initial lesions, whatever their cause, do not appear to cause fatalities *per se*, but act as foci for infection by bacterial and fungal parasites. Evidence supporting this view is based on the observation that the lesions can heal (Fig. 5) if the fish are treated with malachite green to control the development of the fungus (Dunne, 1970; Roberts et al., 1971).

Hume Patterson (1903) was convinced that the "salmon disease" was caused by a bacterium. Subsequently, it has been shown that his *Bacillus Salmonis Pestis* was probably a mixed culture of *Aeromonas liquefaciens* and *Pseudomonas fluorescens* (Bisset, 1946; Carbery, 1968). These bacteria are associated with hemorrhagic septicemia (Wolke, 1975). They are common in freshwater and can be isolated from healthy fish (Collins, 1970). They are now considered to be common facultative fish pathogens, and are not now thought to cause UDN. Nevertheless, the hypothesis that UDN might be caused by a particular species or strain of bacterium is an attractive one and certainly one that warranted investigation. The most serious proposal to come out of these investigations was the suggestion that UDN was caused by a myxobacterium and was, in fact, a cold-water form of "columnaris disease" (Jensen, 1965; Brown, 1966; Brown & Collins, 1966). However, the workers who most forcefully propounded this view later modified their stand (Brown, 1968; Collins & Brown, 1968) and, at present, the weight of the evidence seems contrary to the idea that UDN is caused by a primary bacterial infection.

There is now general agreement that the fungus plays an important role in UDN. Roberts et al. (1971) noted that their ex-

Fig. 5. Completely healed UDN lesions on a salmon (*Salmo salar*) treated with malachite green. (Photograph courtesy of R. J. Roberts, H. J. Ball, A. L. S. Munro, and W. M. Shearer, with permission of The Journal of Fish Biology, Academic Press, Inc. (London) Ltd.)

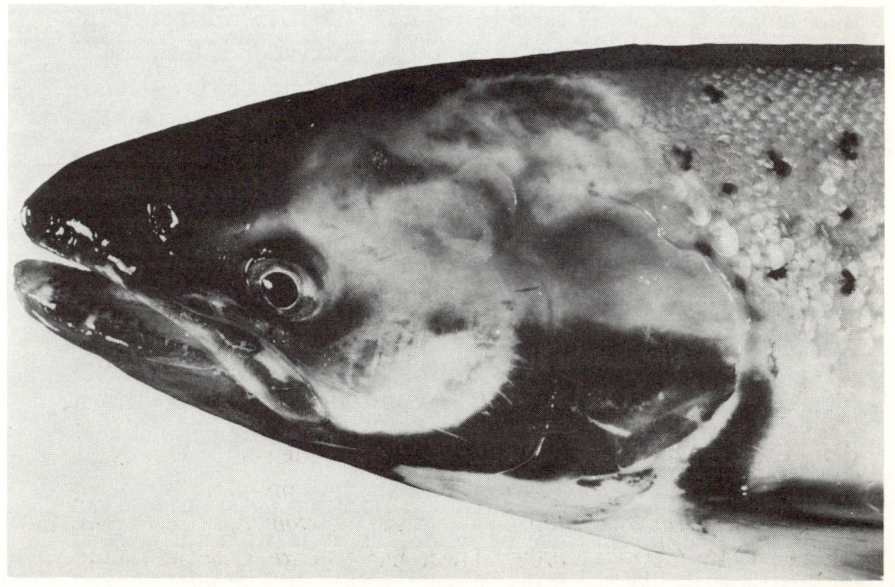

periments indicated " ... the importance of denying access to species of the *Saprolegnia* group of fungi because the establishment of the latter will, in most cases ... result in a fatal outcome." Murphy (1973) noted that ". . . although evidence ascribing a primary etiological role in UDN to fungi is absent there is little doubt that the fungus *Saprolegnia parasitica* [i.e., *Saprolegnia diclina* Type 1] plays an important role in the termination of the disease."

These conclusions reverse the usual trend in dealing with oomycete infections of fishes. There is a strong tendency or, as Bell & Hoskins (1971), tongue-in-cheek, called it, an "article of faith" among hatcherymen and fish pathologists to minimize the role of Oomycetes in fish disease because they are considered to be "secondary invaders" capable of infecting only "debilitated" fish. There is much truth in this notion but, in our opinion, it is not the whole truth and represents an oversimplified viewpoint.

## ON THE NATURE AND CAUSES OF SAPROLEGNIOSIS

As a general rule it may be assumed that saprolegnian fungi are normal and ubiquitous components of freshwater ecosystems and that any body of water capable of supporting fish will not be inimical to these fungi. Coupled with this observation is the parallel observation that most fishes, in most circumstances, do not become infected by these fungi. How then, do we account for the existence of these infections at all? One can approach an answer to this question by proposing two hypotheses. The first hypothesis is that there are specific pathogenic strains of saprolegnian fungi and absence of disease is related to absence of these strains. The second hypothesis is that although the potential host is continuously exposed to potential pathogens it only succumbs to infection when it is debilitated in a way that impairs its normal defences to a degree which allows initiation of the infection. We believe that it is safe to state that the second hypothesis is the more popular and, indeed, the more accurate.

However, in fairness to the pathogenic strain hypothesis, it can be noted that in the case of salmonids at least, there is good evidence that there are specific strains of *Saprolegnia* with a predilection toward parasitism of these fishes. This has been documented by Neish (1976, 1977) for Pacific salmon in Canada (Fig. 6) and by Willoughby (1978) for various British salmonids. Points of similarity between Willoughby's *Saprolegnia diclina* Type 1 and the Category D isolates of Neish (1977) include (1) oogonium production only at "low" temperatures (ca. 5-12°C); (2) poor oogonium production; (3) thin, unpitted oogonial walls (Fig. 6c, f, g); (4) poor oospore production combined with a high rate of oosphere abortion (Fig. 6c, g); (5) relatively small, generally subcentric oospores (Fig. 6e); (6) antheridia of probable diclinous origin (Fig. 6c); and (7) slender antheridia which cover the entire surface of the oogonium (Fig. 6d). The exact degree of similarity between these strains has yet to be established (Willoughby, 1978), as does the relationship between these strains and other *Saprolegnia* isolates belonging to the *S. diclina-S. parasitica* complex which have been isolated from salmonids (Neish, 1976, 1977; Hatai & Egusa, 1977; Hatai, Egusa & Nomura, 1977; Hatai, Egusa & Awakura, 1977).

Peduzzi, Nolard-Tintigner & Bizzozero (1976) and Peduzzi & Bizzozero (1977) have suggested a correlation between the production of a chymotrypsin-like proteolytic enzyme and the capacity for an isolate of *S. ferax* and four isolates in the *S. diclina-S. parasitica* complex to go from a saprotrophic to a necrotrophic mode of nutrition.

Even if one accepts the existence of specific parasitic strains, that there may be seasonal variations in inoculum potential (Suzuki, 1960a, b; Suzuki & Hatekayama, 1961; Hughes, 1962; Roberts, 1963; Hunter, 1975), and that the presence of infected fishes can increase the inoculum potential in a given area (Willoughby & Pickering, 1977), it has not been conclusively demonstrated that fungi known to be parasites of fish in a given watershed (Dudka, 1964; Willoughby, 1969, 1970, 1971; Willoughby & Pickering, 1977) are absent from that watershed at certain times of the year. Therefore a reasonable, if unproven, assumption is that fish are, to a greater or lesser degree, continually challenged by potentially parasitic fungi. As a basic assumption, this holds true even for temperate areas where there may be considerable seasonal variation in water temperature (Neish, 1976). If the environmental conditions are also favorable to infection, one

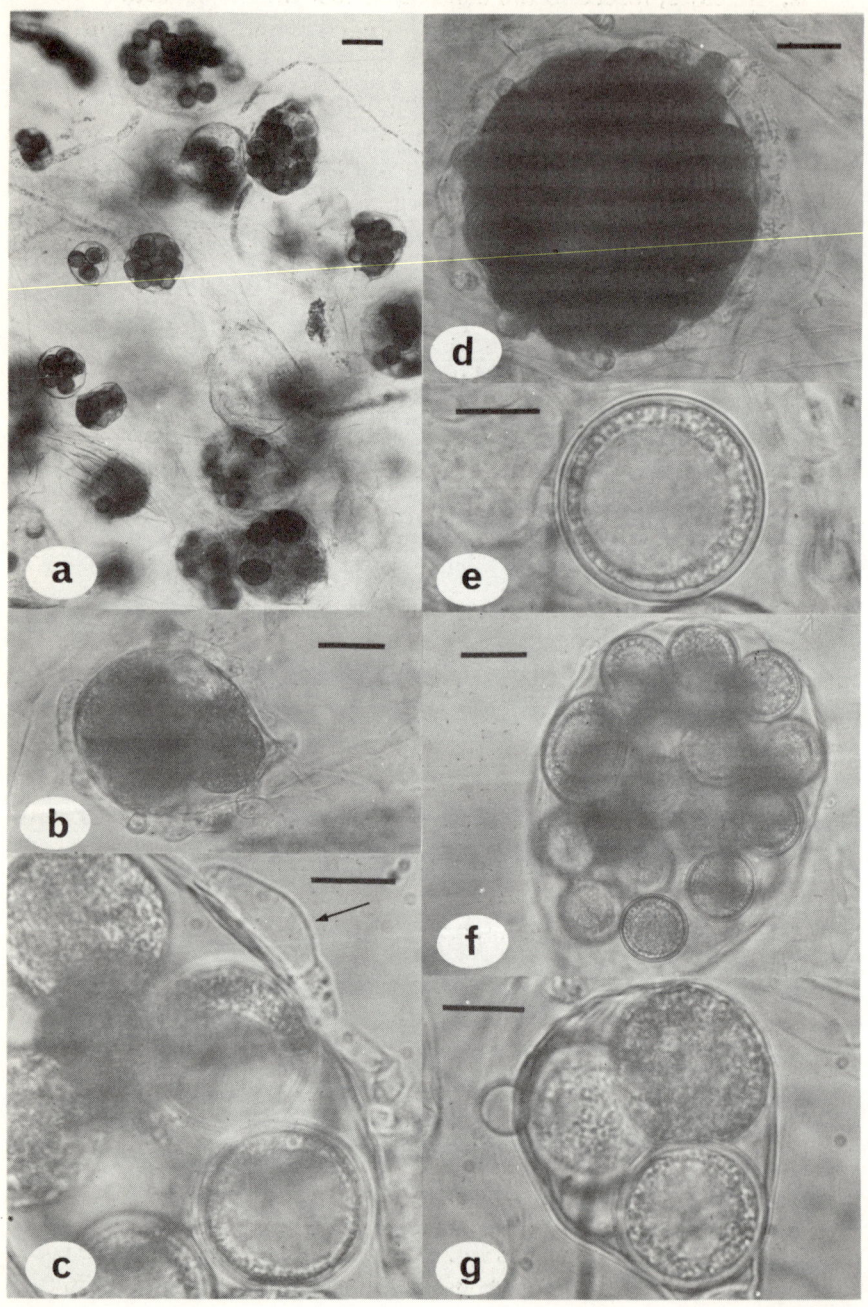

is, therefore, forced to the conclusion that the major factor determining whether an infection is initiated is the condition of the host.

In considering the second hypothesis, we can assert that saprolegnian fungi are "opportunistic" facultative parasites or, using the less ambiguous terminology of Cooke (1977), they are antagonistic facultative symbionts which are necrotrophs when they grow on living organisms and saprotrophs when they derive their nutrition from non-living sources. This is hardly an original conclusion and it has often been used to minimize the importance of saprolegniosis as a disease of fish, instead of recognizing it as the first step toward understanding a complex symbiotic relationship. Many important diseases of fishes, including those caused by some pseudomonads, aeromonads, myxobacteria, and protozoans are caused by "opportunistic" parasites (Robertson et al., 1963; Wedemeyer, 1970; Snieszko, 1974), but for some reason saprolegnian fungi have been singled out as somehow less important than these. For example, if a fish has both an aeromonad infection and a saprolegnian infection, many fish pathologists would regard the aeromonad as the "primary invader" and the fungus as a "secondary invader." This may well be the correct interpretation in many cases, but the danger of this attitude is that it ignores the possibility that, in certain other circumstances, saprolegnian fungi can act as lethal primary pathogens, or as the most serious and destructive pathogen in a mixed infection.

Evidence favouring the idea that saprolegnian fungi can act as primary pathogens is based on controlled infection experiments. The purpose of an infection experiment is to determine whether a

**Opposite:**
Fig. 6. Some morphological features of the *Saprolegnia*, Category D, isolates of Neish (1977). *a*, a cluster of oogonia from a hemp seed culture; *b,c,d,f,g*, oogonia. Note the slender, apparently diclinous antheridia in *b,c,d*, and *g* and the thin oogonial wall best illustrated in *c,f*, and *g*. The arrow in *c* indicates a small, only slightly swollen antheridial cell; *e*, a subcentric oospore. Oospores can also be seen in *c,f*, and *g*. Scale bar = 50 microns for *a*; 20 microns for *b,d*, and *f*; 10 microns for *c,e*, and *g*. (Figs. *6d,e,f*, courtesy of G. A. Neish, with permission of The Journal of Fish Biology, Academic Press, Inc. (London) Ltd.)

particular organism is a potential pathogen. Successful infection experiments help to fulfill Koch's postulates and, at the same time, provide insights into the conditions which will allow the initiation of an infection.

Before an infection experiment using Oomycetes can be considered a success, two criteria must be satisfied. First, the fungus must be observed growing on a living fish and must be seen to invade the living tissue. In other words, its capacity to go from saprotrophy to necrotrophy must be established. If the fungus is found on a dead fish or does not spread beyond necrotic tissue on a living fish, parasitism has not been established. Second, it must be demonstrated that the fungus infecting the fish is the isolate being tested, and not another strain. This second criterion can be difficult to fulfill since it may be difficult to distinguish among related strains; hence re-isolation procedures may not provide definitive results. This problem can be avoided by designing the experiment so that it is reasonable to assume that Oomycetes which could be confused with the strain being tested have been eliminated from the experiment. This can be done by disinfection followed by strict quarantine (O'Bier, 1960; Scott & Warren, 1964; Srivastava, 1976), or by setting up controls so that the only variable is the presence of the test isolate in the experimental tanks (McKay, 1967; Neish, 1976).

As yet, there is no standardized experimental method which will indicate whether or not a given oomycete is a potential fish parasite. Some authors (Hume Patterson, 1903; Rucker, 1944; Egusa, 1965; Egusa & Nishikawa, 1965) have reported that fungal infections will become established only in conjunction with concurrent bacterial infections. Other authors have apparently obtained presumptive primary infections by merely exposing the fish to zoospores of a suspected saprolegnian parasite (Tiffney, 1939b; Hoshina & Ookubo, 1956; Hoshina, Sano & Sunayama, 1960; O'Bier, 1960; Scott & Warren, 1964; McKay, 1967). In most cases, however, these and other authors have reported that it was necessary, or at least desirable, to wound the fish before exposing them to the fungus (Tiffney & Wolf, 1937; Tiffney, 1939b; Hoshina & Ookuba, 1956; Vishniac & Nigrelli, 1957; O'Bier, 1960; Egusa, 1963; Scott & Warren, 1964; Nolard-Tintigner, 1973, 1974; Srivastava, 1976; Srivastava & Srivastava, 1977a, c) and, in some studies (Hoshina & Ookubo, 1956; Nolard-Tintigner, 1973, 1974; Neish, 1976), this has been carried one step further and the wounded area on the fish has been brought into direct contact with the fungal mycelium. In the latter case, however, it should be noted that the best available evidence suggests that the infections are, nonetheless, initiated by spores and not by the hyphae (Nolard-Tintigner, 1973; Willoughby & Pickering, 1977).

Table III gives a list of the species of fish which have succumbed to experimentally induced presumptive primary infections caused by saprolegnian fungi. Even a cursory glance at this table shows that most of these experiments have been restricted to individuals belonging to two closely related genera *(Poecilia, Xiphophorus)* and, excluding these fish, there are few studies which independently confirm and extend the results described in the original reports. Consequently, with the possible exceptions of the Japanese eel *(Anguilla japonica)* and the coho salmon *(Oncorhynchus kisutch)*, surprisingly little is known about the conditions which will permit the establishment of experimentally induced saprolegnian infections in non-cyprinodont fish, including fish which are known to succumb to natural saprolegnian infections and which form the basis of valuable commercial and sport fisheries.

It has often been noted that saprolegnian infections of fish are frequently associated with wounds and lesions and also that handling fish may predispose them to infection. The obvious inference to be drawn from these observations is that these fungi act as "wound parasites"; i.e., that the integument in general and the mucus, in particular, present both a physical and a biochemical barrier to the initiation of infection and that if this barrier can be breached, an infection can proceed unrestrained. This has been discussed in some detail by Wilson (1976) and most recently by Willoughby & Pickering (1977) and Richards & Pickering (1978). These authors have suggested that a reduction in the rate of mucus production, possibly in conjunction with an as yet unclarified decrease in the fungistatic capacity of the mucus, creates a situation which allows the infections to be initiated and accounts for the frequent observation that sexually mature salmonids (similar observations not being available for other fish)

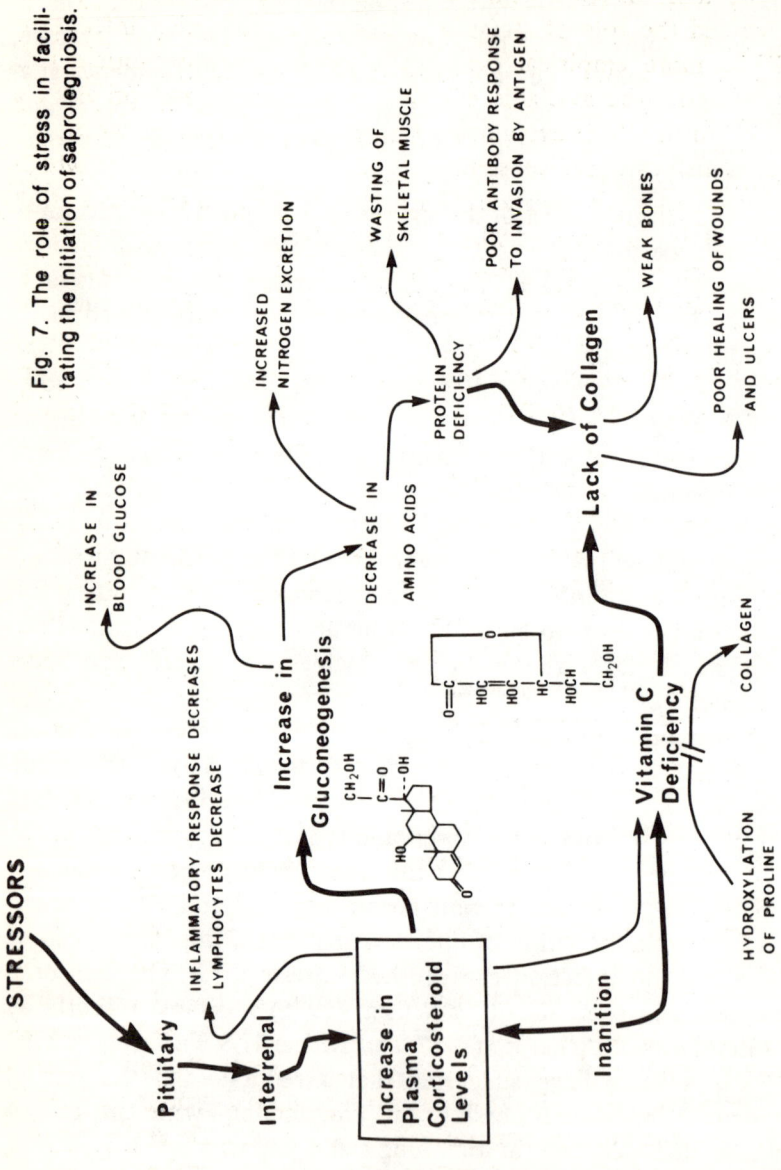

Fig. 7. The role of stress in facilitating the initiation of saprolegniosis.

are more susceptible to infection than immature salmonids.

Based on his work with Pacific salmon, Neish (1976, 1977) emphasized the role of stress in initiating saprolegnian infections. While more empirical evidence is needed to substantiate this hypothesis, the available evidence is persuasive and provides a mechanism which explains how physiological changes which occur in fish can predispose them to infection by parasites to which they are normally resistant. Once again, we should emphasize that most of the evidence on which this hypothesis is based comes from the work with salmonids. This is because the physiology of salmonids seems to be better understood (at least by us) than the physiology of other freshwater fishes. At any rate, having stated our bias, we will present this scheme and hope that it will eventually be shown to have a more universal application. Roth's (1972) work with white suckers (*Catostomus commersonii*) gives us reason to hope that this may indeed prove to be the case.

The basic manner in which the stress response can increase the susceptibility of salmonids to saprolegniosis is shown in Figure 7. This is based, in part, on a similar outline presented by Roddie & Wallace (1975) which is based ultimately on the work of Selye (1950). Wedemeyer (1970) and Wedemeyer, Meyer & Smith (1976) are largely responsible for showing how Selye's stress theory can be applied to fish.

Various stressors, and this could include a variety of both external or internal stimuli acting singly or synergistically, operate through the pituitary-interrenal axis to produce an increase in the level of plasma corticosteroids. Suitable stressors include crowding, injury, suboptimal water temperatures, handling, or the presence of noxious chemicals in sublethal concentrations. A fungal infection itself is also a stressor once it is initiated. An increase in plasma corticosteriod levels can impair the inflammatory responses (McLeay, 1975) and lead to an increase in corticosteroid-regulated protein catabolism and gluconeogenesis (Woodhead, 1975). This can ultimately lead to a protein deficiency which contributes to the wasting of skeletal muscle and leads to a decrease in antibody production and collagen synthesis. Lack of collagen, in turn, impairs the ability of a fish to heal wounds and ulcers.

What we're describing here, of course, is a normal metabolic pathway. The difference which would lead to the initiation of infection is quantitative, not qualitative, and would be associated with periods in the life of a fish during which, for some reason, there were especially high levels of plasma corticosteroids. These periods might be associated with chronic stress such as might be found, for example, in a hatchery where naturally aggressive and territorial fish are crowded together in unnaturally high concentrations. High levels of plasma corticosteroids might also be associated with the fishes' osmoregulatory function (Olivereau, 1962; Utida et al., 1972; Woodhead, 1975), with the necessity to catabolize protein to obtain energy (as, for example, during periods of inanition), or with the inability of fishes to clear the hormone (Woodhead, 1975). In the case of Pacific salmon, periods of especially high corticosteroid levels occur during the downstream migratory period, which is associated with the parr-smolt transformation (McLeay, 1975), and during the upstream migratory period which is associated with sexual maturation (Woodhead, 1975).

Another important (and not unrelated) factor to be considered is the ascorbic acid metabolism of a fish. Fish, in general, have a dietary requirement for Vitamin C, and in the case of salmon this has been well documented (Ashley, Halver & Smith, 1975). In the case of maturing salmon, these reserves become depleted because of inanition and the ability of the fish to repair tissue damage is greatly impaired (Triplett & Calaprice, 1974; Ashley, Halver & Smith, 1975) at a time in their lives when they are quite likely to suffer damage to the integument. Such an explanation does not apply to young salmon, of course, unless they have not had access to an adequate diet, but in this regard it should be noted that an increase in levels of plasma corticosteroids will also cause depletion of ascorbic acid reserves (Wedemeyer, 1969, 1970). Presumably then, even if the salmon are being maintained on a marginally adequate diet, under sufficiently stressful conditions, they could conceivably suffer from a *de facto* ascorbic acid deficiency.

We should emphasize at this point that the stress hypothesis we have presented here is intended to be complementary to the observations of the British workers on mucus production and is not an attempt at an alternative hypothesis. Indeed, there is evidence which suggests that mucus production is controlled by the endocrine system. The main hormone involved in this activity appears to be prolactin, but there is also evidence which does not support this viewpoint (Lam, 1972). Presumably there might be an interaction between prolactin and the interrenal corticosteroids (Utida et al., 1972; Meier, 1972) but, as yet, we are loathe to speculate on the nature of this interaction, or its relation (if any) to the susceptibility of fish to saprolegniosis.

In summary, we believe that there is a direct link between increased plasma corticosteroid levels in fish and their susceptibility to saprolegniosis. These higher hormone levels may occur in response to the physiological requirements of a fish at certain periods in its life (e.g., smoltification, sexual maturation), may be related to stress-induced increases in pituitary-interrenal activity, or come about as a result of both factors acting synergistically. As plasma corticosteroid levels increase, particularly if associated with a period of inanition, the fish become increasingly susceptible to infection and, at the same time, less able to maintain the integrity of their integument. This combination of factors renders them susceptible to infection by saprolegnian fungi and other ubiquitous facultative pathogens. Variation in the stress response of different individuals, species, or populations of fishes to various internal and external stressors at different periods in their lives may well explain, to some extent, a number of the apparently contradictory results obtained by investigators who have carried out infection experiments.

We believe that this stress hypothesis provides a mechanism which shows how saprolegnian fungi may act, on occasion, as primary pathogens and, at the same time, the hypothesis provides a more precise definition of what we mean by a "debilitated" fish. Certainly more empirical evidence is needed to substantiate and elaborate the hypothesis. We have no doubt that further investigation in this area would prove most rewarding.

Parenthetically, we should add that our conception of saprolegniosis is consistent with a much larger body of knowledge relating to mycoses of man and other animals. It is now widely recognized that cortisone therapy, or diseases which interfere with immunocompetency, such as uncontrolled diabetes or leukemia, can predispose a patient to mycoses which are also caused by ubiquitous and normally non-pathogenic fungi—the so-called opportunistic fungal infections (Conant et al., 1971 ; Chick, Balows & Furcolow, 1975).

## PATHOLOGY
### Isolation and Culture of the Parasite

Saprolegnian fungi can be easily isolated from soil or water by using various "baits" such as hemp seeds (Johnson, 1956; Seymour, 1970; Stevens, 1974) or by using various agar media which have been designed for the purpose (Ho, 1975; Willoughby & Pickering, 1977). Isolations from fish or fish eggs can be made by plating mycelium directly onto an agar medium containing a suitable bacteriostatic agent or antibiotics (Neish, 1975b; Willoughby & Pickering, 1977). However, precautions must be taken to ensure that the isolated fungi are the ones actually associated with the lesions. The foremost precaution is to ensure, whenever possible, that the mycelium is obtained from a living or freshly killed fish. This reduces the risk of isolating purely saprotrophic contaminants. Records of saprolegnian fungi from dead fishes or fish eggs cannot be regarded as parasites in the absence of confirmation from controlled infection experiments.

Even when an isolate is obtained from a living or freshly killed fish and plated out onto nutrient agar, theoretically, competitive effects could inhibit the growth of the true pathogen while more aggressive saprotrophic fungi could become dominant. This is why it is desirable to examine the lesions to observe the morphological forms present as soon as possible after the isolations have been made. Willoughby (1978) has described a procedure where portions of lesions are examined for several days to observe the forms that develop.

Finally, even when all precautions have been taken, single spore isolates should be obtained from the original cultures and these isolates should be tested in infection experiments using the same species (or at least the same genus) of fish from which they were originally obtained. This, as noted previously, has only been done a few times. In carrying out such infection experiments, it must be remembered that negative results do not prove that the isolate is *not* a pathogen.

The foregoing are, to a certain extent, theoretical considerations. In practice, at least for salmonids, it appears that a sufficient number of isolations from freshly killed fish give an accurate picture of the fungi actually involved in the lesions (Neish, 1977; Willoughby, 1978). We suspect that this is due to the fact that the *Saprolegnia* species isolated from these fish are as aggressive as saprotrophs as they are as necrotrophs. Also, present evidence indicates that these lesions tend to be unifungal. These circumstances are not, however, universally true and more work and new innovative approaches are needed in this area.

### Gross Pathology

Infections caused by Oomycetes form a cottony, white growth on fish and fish eggs (Plates 1-5) putting them among the easiest of all fish diseases to diagnose. The colour of the mycelium can vary from white, depending on the colour of the particles which get trapped in the mycelium. Often, because of the presence of sediment particles, the mycelium has a brownish colour. Microscopic examination of the mycelium from the lesions will reveal the characteristic transparent, coenocytic mycelium (Fig. 8), and usually numerous sporangia will be present. If sporangia are present, one can often make a tentative generic identification. For the purposes of treatment, diagnosis need generally proceed no further since the same chemotherapeutic and chemoprophylactic measures are used for all Oomycetes. However, it must be borne in mind that other infections (viral, bacterial, protozoan), less easy to diagnose, might also be present and that the occurrence of a saprolegnian infection can mask the characteristic signs and symptoms of these diseases as, for example, in the frequent cases where there is concurrent occurrence of saprolegnian and bacterial septicemic infections.

Saprolegnian infections of fish, once initiated, generally tend to be progressive and terminal. The mycelium spreads outward from the initial focus of infection and adjacent infections become confluent. As the infection progresses the fish usually becomes increasingly lethargic; it tires more easily and becomes less responsive to external stimuli. The presence of light colored fungal patches makes the fish more conspicuous, and the mycelium can offer physical resistance to the passage of the fish through the water. Obviously a fish in this condition is an easy target for predators. Loss of equilibrium often occurs shortly before death.

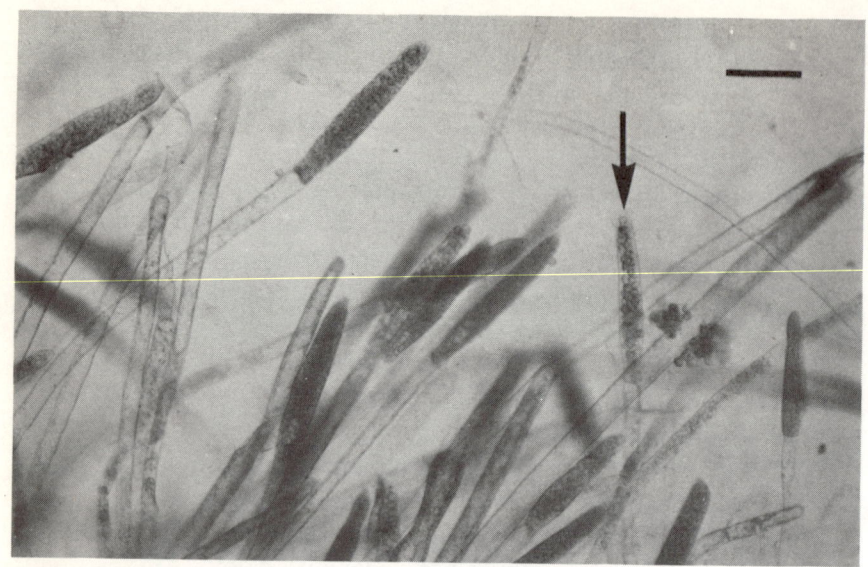

Fig. 8. Water mount of mycelium of *Saprolegnia* sp. removed directly from an infected salmon (*Oncorhynchus* sp.). Arrow indicates a zoosporangium releasing zoospores through an atypical lateral exit papilla. Scale bar = 10 microns. (With permission of The Journal of Fish Biology, Academic Press, Inc. (London) Ltd.)

Temperature can have a marked effect on the initiation and subsequent development of the lesions. However, there is no pat formula as to what this effect might be and more experimental work needs to be done in this area. Work in our laboratory (McKay, 1967; Neish, 1976) with young coho salmon has shown that lower temperatures favour the host over the parasite and can retard the rate of initiation and development of the infections. In one experiment, for example, Neish (1976) found that fish maintained at 7°C survived about three times longer than fish maintained at 17°C before succumbing to the infections. This finding is consistent with the observation that both hyphal growth and zoospore production by the fungus decrease with decreasing temperature and, at the same time, lower temperatures presumably favour the hosts since they are coldwater fish (Brett, Shelbourn & Shoop, 1969).

Virtually any area on the surface of a fish may become infected. Usually it is the integument which is involved (Plates 1-4), but the gills (Plate 13), eyes (Plate 10), and olfactory pits may also become infected. Also, as noted previously, there are rare reports of infections being initiated in the gut.

For a particular disease outbreak, one would not generally expect the lesions to occur at random but to occur in specific patterns or locations. In some cases this may be a result of the fact that specific types of wounds or lesions that act as foci of infection occur in specific locations; for example, on the head of an Atlantic salmon with UDN. Another example would be the caudal peduncle of young salmonids. This area can become infected in subordinate fish because of "tail nipping" activity by the dominant fish. The combination of stress and injury allows initiation of the infection.

In other cases, the lesions occur in distinct patterns or locations but the reasons for the patterning are more obscure. Richards & Pickering (1978) reported a sexual difference in both the pattern and incidence of infection in sexually mature brown trout and White (1975) also reported a similar sexual difference in the pattern of infection in that species. This difference was related to sexual dimorphism in the structure of the skin with relation to a reduction in the number of goblet cells. McKay (1967) and Neish (1976, 1977) have discussed patterns of infection in young and sexually mature oncorhynchids respectively. Hatai, Egusa & Nomura (1977) have discussed patterns of infection in juvenile rainbow trout. In eastern Europe there is a characteristic saprolegniosis of the olfactory pits of carp known as "Staff's disease" (Bauer, Musselius & Strelkov, 1973).

The frequent observation that saprolegnian fungi colonize dead eggs and then proceed to smother adjacent living eggs is, in our experience, quite accurate. Given the nature of modern hatchery operations, it seems safe to say that without some form of intervention (usually through chemoprophylaxis or by manual removal of dead eggs) the vast majority of embryos would never hatch.

## Histopathology

The two most popular techniques for demonstrating saprolegnian fungi in fish tissues are Grocott's (1955) methenamine-silver method (Bucke, 1972; Nolard-Tintigner, 1973, 1974; Bootsma,

1973; Wolke, 1975) and the periodic acid-Schiff's technique used in conjunction with a light green counterstain (PAS-light green) (Roberts et al., 1969, 1970; Neish, 1977). Using the Grocott technique the hyphae stain brown to black (Plates 9-11) whereas with PAS they stain pink to red (Plates 7, 8, 13). In the tissues, the hyphae appear as coenocytic, irregularly branched structures and show no departure from their normal morphology to indicate that a necrotrophic mode of nutrition has any influence on the morphology of the vegetative mycelium.

Tissue to be examined histologically should be fixed as soon as possible after the death of the fish to avoid post mortem growth of the hyphae. Popular fixatives are Bouin's and 10% neutral buffered formalin. Bucke (1972) has provided guidelines for histological procedures applicable to fish tissues.

Generally, as noted previously, saprolegnian infections are associated with the integument and can cause rapid destruction of the epidermis, thus depriving the fish of the protection of the mucus. Penetration by the hyphae through the basement membrane and into the dermis further compromises the integrity of the integument. Compare, for example, Plate 6 with Plate 7. In cases where saprolgenian infections are restricted to the integument, it seems reasonable to suppose that the actual cause of death may be related to impaired osmoregulation and the inability of the fish to maintain its body-fluid balance (Gardner, 1974; Hargens & Perez, 1975). In the case of destruction of the gill tissues (Plates 12, 13) these effects would, of course, be exacerbated by the impaired respiration.

An important point to stress, however, is that saprolegnian fungi are not tissue specific and are capable of attacking virtually any tissue (Plates 6-13). This aspect has been most carefully documented in the detailed studies of Nolard-Tintigner (1973, 1974) but various other studies have extended and confirmed the general applicability of these observations (Bootsma, 1973; Dukes, 1975; Wolke, 1975; Neish, 1977; Hatai & Egusa, 1977). Hence the common designation of saprolegniosis as a "dermatomycosis" is both inaccurate and misleading. This perception probably arises as a result of the fact that these infections are usually initiated in the integument followed by the fish's death before the infecting fungus can proceed beyond the integument or the underlying musculature.

It appears that, in general, the inflammatory response of the fish to saprolegniosis is, as Wolke (1975) put it, "surprisingly slight." Wolke (1975) noted lymphocytic and macrophagic infiltration of the musculature whereas Nolard-Tintigner (1973) reported that histiocytes were the main inflammatory cells in the musculature and monocytes were the main inflammatory cells in the circulatory system. Bootsma (1973) found no inflammatory cells and Nolard-Tintigner (1973) reported that in about 20% of the fish she examined, there was no inflammatory response in the musculature. With regard to primary saprolegniosis, presence or absence of inflammatory cells appears to have no effect on the progress of the infection.

The results of histopathological studies of natural infections must be regarded critically with a view toward understanding the combined effects of mixed infections. Wolke (1975), for example, discussed this with relation to leukocytotoxin production by *Aeromonas salmonicida*.

It does not appear likely that saprolegnian fungi produce any toxins (Rucker, 1944; Nolard-Tintigner, 1973; Peduzzi, Nolard-Tintigner & Bizzozero, 1976). The damage done by these fungi can be directly related to tissue necrosis in the immediate area of the hyphae. Assuming that the fungus is the only pathogen, the time of death will be a function of the growth rate of the fungus, the initial site of infection, the type and quantity of tissue destroyed, and the ability of the individual fish to withstand the stress of the disease.

## PREVENTION AND TREATMENT

Prevention and treatment of saprolegnian infections of fishes and fish eggs have attracted a lot of attention for a long time and a vast array of chemicals has been tested for effectiveness against these fungi *in vitro* (Scott & Warren, 1964; Hodkinson & Hunter, 1970; Bootsma, 1973; Srivastava, 1976) and *in vivo* (Hoffman & Meyer, 1974). A comprehensive, but by no means exhaustive, list of these chemicals includes acriflavine, collargol, copper sulfate, diquat, formalin, gentian violet (crystal violet), griseofulvin, a gardinol type detergent (Teepol), hydroquinone, malachite green, merbromin (Mercurochrome), neutral red, nifurpirinol (Furanace), ozone, 2-phenoxyethanol, potassium chromate, potassium dichromate, potassium permanganate, sodium chloride, and silver nitrate (Hoffman & Meyer, 1974; Srivastava, 1976). It has even been suggested that a cure could be effected by dipping fish into asphalt (Behler, as cited by Ryder, 1883)! In addition to chemical prophylaxis and treatment, ultraviolet irradiation (Kokhanskaya, 1973) and biological control using bacteria (Mazilkin, 1957) or crustaceans (Oseid, 1977) have been used in attempts to prevent and control saprolegniosis of fish eggs.

Despite the fact that it is a potential mutagen, carcinogen, and teratogen (Steffens et al., 1961; Glagoleva & Malikova, 1968; Nelson, 1974) and its use has been curtailed in the USSR (Bauer, Musselius & Strelkov, 1973), zinc-free malachite green is probably the most popular agent for controlling saprolegniosis. The popularity of this chemical stems from the fact that it is an inexpensive and effective fungicide and, in general, allows a wide margin of error between therapeutic and toxic dosages. Nelson (1974) has provided a comprehensive review of the literature concerning the use of malachite green in fisheries and information on the practical application of this chemical can be found in Hoffman & Meyer (1974), Wood (1974), and Roberts & Shepherd (1974). Dosages in the range of 1-5 mg per liter are generally used for bath or flush treatments, 67 mg per liter for short dips, and topical applications at dosages as high as 100,000 mg per liter have been used for treating salmon (Plate 14).

Formalin is also an inexpensive and popular chemoprophylactic and chemotherapeutic agent. Literature concerned with its use in fisheries biology has been recently reviewed by Schnick (1973). Practical information on the application of formalin can be found in Rucker (1963), Schnick (1973), Wood (1974), Hoffman & Meyer (1974), and Roberts & Shepherd (1974). When using formalin, contamination with paraformaldehyde must be avoided and special care must be taken to ensure thorough mixing.

Although malachite green and formalin are both popular and widely used, neither of them can be considered an ideal therapeutant, and we hope that research will continue on the development of safer alternatives. In this regard, we feel that perhaps common salt (NaCl) has not been given the attention it deserves as a chemotherapeutant despite the fact that it is inexpensive, safe, and apparently efficacious (Davis, 1953) at concentrations of about 30,000 mg per liter. Also, novel approaches such as Oseid's (1977) use of the isopod *Asellus militaris* may provide a means of controlling the proliferation of fungi while permitting a reduction in the use of fungicides, most of whose effects on the environment, fishes, or man are not fully understood.

# BRANCHIOMYCES

## SYSTEMATICS, PATHOLOGY AND EPIZOOTIOLOGY

Branchiomycosis (gill rot, Kiemenfäule) was first recognized by the pioneer fish pathologist Marianne Plehn who described *Branchiomyces sanguinis* Plehn as a parasite of carp *(Cyprinus carpio)* at the Munich Biological Research Station during the summer of 1911 (Plehn, 1912, 1924). Further reports by Scheuring & Walter (1926) and Scheuring & Gaschott (1928) followed by the detailed studies by Schäperclaus (1929) and Wundsch (1929, 1930) extended these observations. Wundsch (1929, 1930) described a second species, *Branchiomyces demigrans* Wundsch as a parasite of pike *(Esox lucius)* and tench *(Tinca tinca)*. These early investigations in Germany, and later studies in other areas in Europe, led to what might be called the "standard" description of branchiomycosis as presented by Schäperclaus (1954), Keiz (1959), Bartsch (1968), Amlacher (1970), Reichenbach-Klinke (1973) and others. According to this description, branchiomycosis can be divided into two relatively distinct entities as follows:

1. branchiomycosis of carp (but also including tench, *Carassius auratus gibelio* and sticklebacks) caused by *Branchiomyces sanguinis* (Plate 15).
2. branchiomycosis of pike and tench caused by *Branchiomyces demigrans*.

Both species of *Branchiomyces* are known only as parasites of gill tissues and both species produce branched coenocytic hyphae capable of producing aplanospores by endogenous cleavage (Plates 16-18). The two species are separated by differences in morphology and characteristic growth habit as summarized in Table IV. The key diagnostic features used for the separation of the species are the thicker hyphal walls, somewhat larger spores, and extravascular growth attributed to *B. demigrans* (hence the specific epithet, derived from the Latin verb *demigrare* = to emigrate).

The differences between the two species are probably not as distinct as Table IV suggests. Bespalyi (1950) was convinced that he had observed both forms in a single culture maintained in blood broth and more recently this problem has been reviewed by Lucký (1970) who notes that there is evidence which indicates that the criteria used for separating the two species may be more indicative of the variation of a single species in response to different hosts and environments. Grimaldi et al. (1973), in their extensive study of *Branchiomyces* infections of fishes from lakes in Italy and Switzerland, were not able to assign the form they examined to either species with confidence.

To solve a problem of this type, the classical microbiological approach is to establish pure cultures of the organisms in question and compare them in various ways under controlled conditions. This is difficult if the organisms in question are so fastidious that much effort must be expended to establish cultures, but this situation does not appear to apply to *Branchiomyces* species. Bespalyi (1950) was apparently able to establish cultures in blood broth with relative ease and Apizidi (1959) found that *B. sanguinis* grew well in a medium containing 10% duck excrement decoction, 10 % gelatin, and 0.1% citric acid with pH adjusted to 5.8. More recently, Dankó, Szabó & Szakolczai (1967) and Peduzzi (1973) have been able to grow *Branchiomyces* isolates on routine agar media commonly found in mycology laboratories. Given the apparent ease with which these cultures were established, and the intrinsic mycological, biological, and economic importance of *Branchiomyces* species, it seems curious to us that these organisms have not attracted more attention from mycologists. Moreover, despite the ease with which cultures can apparently be maintained and transferred, it appears that no cultures have ever been deposited in a culture collection.

The descriptions of *Branchiomyces* isolates in culture presented by Dankó, Szabó & Szakolczai (1967) and Peduzzi (1973) would have been helped by more thorough illustration, but in general, it appears that the appearance of *Branchiomyces* in culture is similar to its appearance in the gills of infected fish (Fig. 9). According to Dankó, Szabó & Szakolczai (1967), about a week after inoculation thin, brown, pellicle-like colonies can be seen on the surface of Sabouraud's maltose agar. The hyphae apparently just lie on the

## Table IV

**Diagnostic features used for the separation of *Branchiomyces sanguinis* from *Branchiomyces demigrans* (based on Schäperclaus, 1954; Amlacher, 1970 and others).**

|  | *B. sanguinis* | *B. demigrans* |
|---|---|---|
| Principal Host | *Cyprinus carpio* | *Esox lucius*<br>*Tinca tinca* |
| Occurrence | Usually localized in the blood vessels of the gill arch, gill filaments and lamellae | Hyphae can penetrate the gill filament and occur on the surface of the filament. |
| Morphometric Comparisons |  |  |
| hyphal diameter | 8-30 microns | Usually 13-14 microns; up to 22-28 microns at the tips |
| hyphal wall thickness | ca. 0.2 microns | 0.5-0.7 microns |
| spore diameter | 5-9 microns | 12-17 microns |

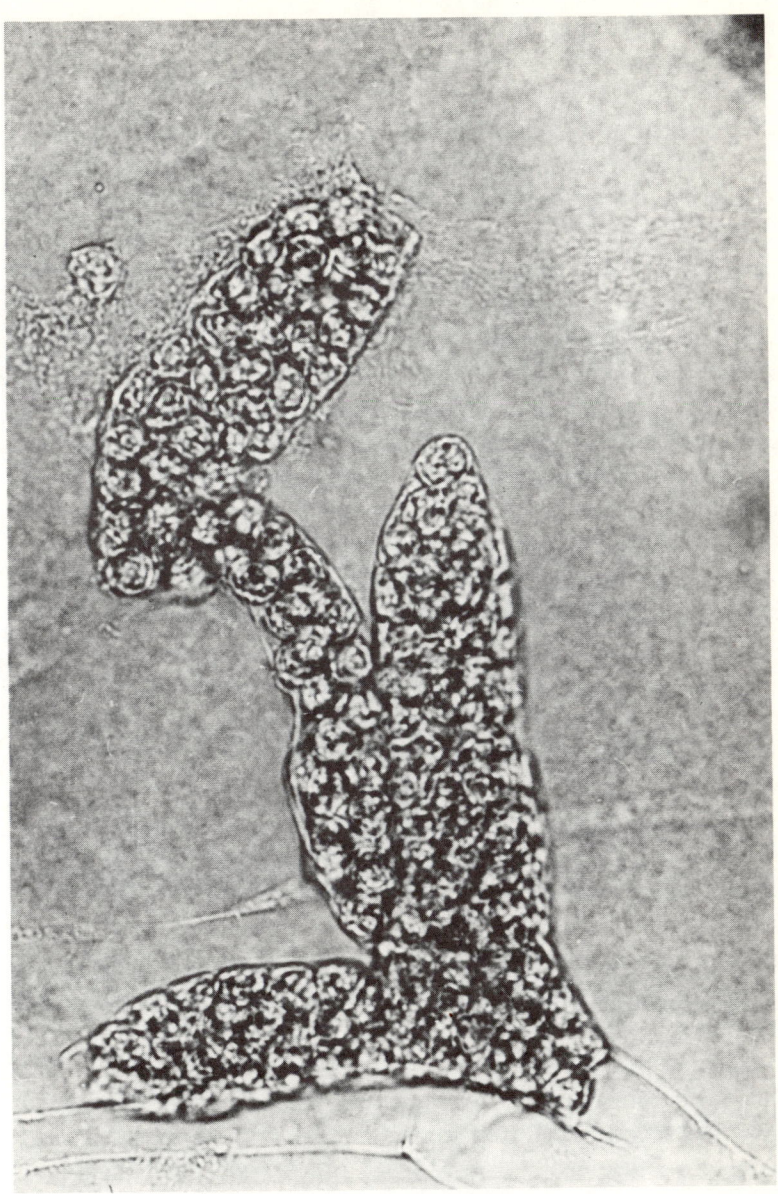

Fig. 9. Squash preparation in water of a culture obtained from a bleak from Lake di Annone, Italy, infected by *Branchiomyces* sp. Grown on gill extract angar. X 600. (Photograph courtesy of Peduzzi, Meng & Polli.)

surface of the agar and produce neither aerial nor submerged hyphae. Spores were produced in the older hyphae and the dimensions of the spores and hyphae were the same as those seen in the fish. Peduzzi (1973) apparently found sporangia and, on hemp seeds, gemmae. It is difficult, however, to compare Peduzzi's (1973) isolate with the isolate studied by Dankó, Szabó & Szakolczai (1967) simply on the basis of their published descriptions. We get the impression that these cultures may have differed in some respects with regard to morphology and growth habit.

Peduzzi (1973) was able to show that the antigenic structure of his *Branchiomyces* isolate was very similar to that of four different *Saprolegnia* isolates and this, combined with the morphological features of *Branchiomyces*, led him to suggest that this genus may belong in the Saprolegniaceae. It would be most interesting if this suggestion could be supported by further evidence and readily available cultures.

Branchiomycosis has, until recently, been regarded as a disease which has a relatively limited host range and geographic distribution, and also as a disease which occurs within a relatively narrowly defined set of environmental parameters (Schäperclaus, 1954; Amlacher, 1970; Bauer, Musselius & Strelkov, 1973). Hence, a "typical" outbreak would be one affecting two- or three-year-old carp being maintained in a pond somewhere in eastern Europe (e.g., southern Poland, Czechoslovakia, Hungary, Yugoslavia, the Ukraine). This pond would be highly enriched with nitrogenous organic compounds resulting, for example, from the addition of various types of manure to the water to increase fertility. The outbreak would occur during the warmest months of the year (July, August), often after a warm spell, when the water temperature was in excess of 20°C.

In recent years, however, it has become increasingly clear that although, from both an economic and epizootiologic standpoint, banchiomycosis is still most important as a disease of pond fishes in eastern Europe, the disease has a much wider host range and geographic distribution than previously suspected. According to Sarig (1971), branchiomycosis is known in Israel and other countries bordering the Mediterranean. Hora & Pillay (1962) noted that branchiomycosis is fairly common among cultivated fishes in the Indo-Pacific region and Egusa & Ohiwa (1972) have presented a well documented case of branchiomycosis among pond-reared eels (*Anguilla japonica*) in Japan. Meyer & Robinson (1973) and Wolke (1975) have found branchiomycosis in a total of five species of fishes from ponds in Arkansas and Rhode Island in the eastern United States. Grimaldi et al. (1973) have considerably extended the known host range of branchiomycosis in western Europe in work that was initiated after Grimaldi (1971) discovered an epizootic of bleak (*Alburnus alburnus alborella*) in Lake Maggiore in northern Italy caused by a *Branchiomyces* species. Extension of this work to other fish species and other lakes in Italy and Switzerland showed that some degree of infection could be demonstrated in 21 of 24 species examined. These records, along with other records known to us, are shown in Table V.

The work by Grimaldi (1971) and Grimaldi et al. (1973) further established two other important points. First, these authors demonstrated that branchiomycosis was present in large, deep lakes as well as in small, warm, highly eutrophic ponds or lakes. Second, they demonstrated that chronic infections could be present in numerous fish species not known to suffer from epizootics caused by *Branchiomyces*. These findings force a radical departure from the traditional ideas concerning branchiomycosis, and one has to wonder if the rapid extension of the host range and geographic distribution over the past decade is due to an actual increase in the incidence of infection or to an increase in the incidence of alert fish pathologists.

Grimaldi et al. (1973) have suggested that increased eutrophication of some lakes has encouraged the development of pathogenic strains of *Branchiomyces* and, at the same time, has encouraged the proliferation of cyprinids, the group of fish most susceptible to infection, with *Alburnus* species in this case being the most seriously afflicted. They go on to suggest that the contagion can then be spread to less eutrophic lakes by way of hydrologic connections. As partial support of this hypothesis they noted that no evidence of branchiomycosis could be found in the fish populations of some oligotrophic lakes in Switzerland which are hydrographically separate from the nearby lakes in northern Italy. More recently, Giussani, Borroni & Grimaldi (1976) have discussed the potential role of temperature and un-ionized ammonia as factors predisposing bleak to infection in Lake Maggiore. They found a correlation

## Table V
### Species of fishes reported to be susceptible to branchiomycosis

| Species[1] | References |
|---|---|
| **ANGUILLIDAE** | |
| *Anguilla anguilla* | Grimaldi et al., 1973 |
| *Anguilla japonica* | Egusa & Ohiwa, 1972 |
| **ATHERINIDAE** | |
| *Atherina boyeri* (= *A. mochon*) | Grimaldi et al., 1973 |
| **CENTRARCHIDAE** | |
| *Micropterus dolomieui* | Meyer & Robinson, 1973 |
| *Micropterus salmoides* | Meyer & Robinson, 1973; Grimaldi et al., 1973 |
| *Lepomis gibbosus* | Grimaldi et al., 1973; Wolke, 1975 |
| *Lepomis macrochirus* | Wolke, 1975 |
| **COBITIDAE** | |
| *Cobitis taenia* | Grimaldi et al., 1973 |
| *Coregonus* spp. | Radulescu, Vasiliu-Suceveanu & Luscan, 1957; Einsele, 1959; Lopukhina, 1959; Tesarcík & Hoska, 1962; Tesarcík, Smísek & Hluzek, 1965; Rehulka & Tesarcík, 1972; Grimaldi et al., 1973 |
| *Coregonus albula* | Huculak, 1958 |
| **CYPRINIDAE** | |
| *Alburnus albidus* (= *Alburnus alburnus alborella*) | Grimaldi, 1971; Grimaldi et al., 1973 |
| *Carassius auratus gibelio* | Heuschmann, 1935; Schäperclaus, 1954 |
| *Carassius carassius* | Shcherbina, 1960 |
| *Chondrostoma soëtta* | Grimaldi et al., 1973 |
| *Cyprinus carpio* | Plehn, 1912; Scheuring & Walter, 1926; Scheuring & Gaschott, 1928; Schäperclaus, 1929, 1954; Volf, 1933; Bespalyi, 1949, 1950; Ivasik & Demchenko, 1959; Shcherbina, 1960; Rehulka & Tesarcik; 1972; and numerous other reports. |
| *Gobio gobio* | Scerban, 1954 |
| *Leuciscus cephalus* | Grimaldi et al., 1973 |
| *Rutilus pigus* | Grimaldi et al., 1973 |
| *Scardinius erythrophthalmus* | Grimaldi et al., 1973 |

[1] Since most of the records reported here are from Europe, we have followed the nomenclature of Blanc et al. (1971) for the most part.

| Species | References |
|---|---|
| *Tinca tinca* | Wundsch, 1929; Rehulka & Tesarcík, 1972; Grimaldi et al., 1973 |
| **ESOCIDAE** | |
| *Esox lucius* | Wundsch, 1929, 1930; Volf, 1956; Grimaldi et al., 1973 |
| **GADIDAE** | |
| *Lota lota* | Grimaldi et al., 1973 |
| **GASTEROSTEIDAE** | |
| *Gasterosteus aculeatus* | Schäperclaus, 1954 |
| **ICTALURIDAE** | |
| *Ictalurus melas* | Grimaldi et al., 1973 |
| **PERCIDAE** | |
| *Perca fluviatilis* | Grimaldi et al., 1973 |
| **SALMONIDAE** | |
| *Salmo gairdneri* | Tománek, 1962; Barthelmes, Mattheis & Meyer, 1968; Witala & Zielonka, 1974 |
| *Salmo trutta* | Grimaldi et al., 1973 |
| *Salvelinus alpinus* | Grimaldi et al., 1973 |
| **SILURIDAE** | |
| *Siluris glanis* | Dankó, Szabó, & Szakolczai, 1967; Lucký, 1970 |

between increased temperature (20.5-25.5 °C) and a sharp increase of un-ionized ammonia (up to 10 ppb) and the incidence of branchiomycosis. A sharp increase in un-ionized ammonia in the spring, when the water temperature was between 10-14 °C, was correlated with what appeared to be an outbreak of bacterial gill disease but there was no evidence of *Branchiomyces*.

Branchiomycosis can appear suddenly and often has a rapid course with losses as high as 30-50% occurring in 2-4 days. Death is due to anoxia and infected fishes become quite listless. There is some disagreement about other gross symptoms of the disease. For example, Bauer, Musselius & Strelkov (1973) stated that the fish do not swallow air when they have the disease, but Amlacher (1970) and Meyer & Robinson (1973) both noted that infected fish exhibit obvious respiratory distress.

Not all species of fishes in an affected pond necessarily become infected, even if they are known suscepts. Dankó, Szabó & Szakolczai (1967) reported heavy losses of *Siluris glanis* while carp, tench and silver carp (*Hypophthalmichthys molotrix*) being maintained in the same ponds were unaffected.

In *Branchiomyces* infections the fungal hyphae obstruct the circulation of blood through the gills and the infected areas lose their normal bright red color and instead exhibit brownish areas due to hemorrhage and thrombosis and lighter whitish or greyish areas as a result of ischemia (Plate 15). This gives the gills a "marbled" appearance which is considered to be pathognomonic for acute branchiomycosis (Rehulka & Tesarcík, 1972; Bauer, Musselius & Strelkov, 1973). Microscopically, proliferation of the lamellar epithelial cells and lamellar fusion may be observed in addition to necrosis of the infected tissues (Plate 16). The necrotic areas may slough off and these areas can also become a focus for saprolegnian infections; however, not all infected fish die and these fish can recover and eventually regenerate the lost tissue.

There appear to be differences in the inflammatory response. Meyer & Robinson (1973) reported that the fish did not show a marked inflammatory response and they found no invasion of leucocytes in the affected area. Dankó, Szabó & Szakolczai (1967), on the other hand, reported that they usually observed a leucocytic inflammatory response. Bespalyi (1950) found an increase in granulocytes, monocytes and polymorphonuclear leucocytes and a marked reduction in the lymphocyte count.

It is not known exactly what the reservoir of infection is, how the infections are initiated, or whether the infections can be spread from fish to fish. It is usually assumed that the fungus occurs as a saprobe in nature but, to our knowledge, this organism has never been isolated from any natural source other than the gills of a fish. Since *Branchiomyces* isolates apparently grow relatively easily in culture, it is interesting that an isolate has never been picked up during the course of the many investigations of fungi from freshwater habitats. Perhaps part of the problem might rest with the failure of mycologists to recognize the fungus. It is also usually assumed that the aplanospores produced by the fungus can act as a source of contagion but this does not appear to have been verified experimentally and there appears to be no information regarding the germination of these spores. Peduzzi (1973) obtained a successful infection of a bleak by inoculating mycelium onto the gill arch with a microspatula, but the exact manner in which the infection was initiated was not studied. It was noted by Amlacher (1970) that *Branchiomyces* species preferentially attack the efferent branchial arteries whereas Grimaldi et al. (1973) found that in different species of fish, different areas of the branchial arch are attacked, yielding patterns which appear to be specific for each species of fish.

## PREVENTION AND TREATMENT

Various chemicals have been used to treat branchiomycosis. Dankó, Szabó & Szakolczai (1967) reported successful treatment of *Silurus glanis* by maintaining fish in 0.3 mg per liter malachite green for 24 hours. Huet (1972) recommends a one hour bath containing 1-4 ppm active ingredient of benzalkonium chloride or 100 mg per liter copper sulfate for 10-30 minutes. Meyer & Robinson (1973) found that continuous baths containing 0.5 mg per liter copper sulfate or 0.1 mg per liter malachite green were toxic, but some success was obtained with initial treatments of 15 ppm formalin followed by subsequent and repeated applications at 25 ppm. Other workers (Alikuhni, 1957; Shcherbina, 1952) have recommended salt baths of 3-5% for prophylaxis and control. However, the efficacy of these treatments is not well established nor, for that matter, the dose, which is dependent on water quality and hardness and on the species, age, and condition of the affected fish. In any case, the generally sudden onset and rapid course of branchiomycosis would most likely lead to a high mortality before treatment could be instituted. For these reasons, most attempts to control branchiomycosis are, quite properly, directed toward prevention rather than treatment.

Reichle (1973) suggested feeding methylene blue to fish with branchiomycosis, particularly when the disease is accompanied by secondary infections. Since methylene blue is known to effect significant increases in haemoglobin content (Tack, 1960) and erythrocyte count (Reichenbach-Klinke, 1975), it seems to us that this procedure is worthy of further investigation.

Preventive measures are based on the elimination of those environmental factors which are thought to encourage the initiation of infection. Basically, these measures consist of taking steps to prevent the water from becoming too warm and to prevent the excessive accumulation of decomposing organic matter in the ponds during the critical warm months of the year. These goals are accomplished by increasing the water exchange in the ponds, controlling the addition of fertilizer to the ponds, reducing the amount of food given to the fish, and by controlling the number of waterfowl allowed on the ponds.

Chemoprophylactic measures include the addition of copper sulfate as an algicide, and the addition of quicklime (CaO) to raise the pH and help clarify the water. According to Schäperclaus (1954), a total of 8 kg per hectare copper sulfate should be added to ponds with an average depth of 0.5 m and a total of 12 kg per hectare to ponds with an average depth of 1.0 m. The copper sulfate is added in four treatments of two or three kg per hectare respectively at monthly intervals starting in mid-May and ending in mid-August. This procedure can yield initial concentrations of 0.3-0.4 mg per liter if properly applied, and this concentration should be tolerated by most fishes and is within the tolerance level of 1.0 ppm allowed by the U.S. Environmental Protection Agency for potable waters. However, it must be remembered that copper is quite toxic for many aquatic organisms and that the effective and safe dosage depends very much on the water quality and the species of fish being treated. As with all chemoprophylactic procedures, copper sulfate should not be used promiscuously and readers are encouraged to refer to the literature review by Jackson (1974) on the use of copper sulfate and to also note the comments by Gardner & LaRoche (1973) and Reichenbach-Klinke (1975) concerning the effects of copper sulfate on fish. In this regard, it is worth noting that Reichenbach-Klinke (1975) strongly discourages use of copper salts in fish culture except in critical situations.

The use of lime in fisheries has been recently reviewed by Sills (1974). Bauer, Musselius & Strelkov (1973) recommend the introduction of 150-200 kg quicklime (CaO) per hectare into ponds affected by branchiomycosis. This is added at two-week intervals during the summer and daily during an outbreak. The pH should be monitored and should not be allowed to exceed 9.0 (Schäperclaus, 1954).

If an outbreak occurs, feeding of the fish should be stopped and dead fish should be removed from the ponds and buried in a lime pit. To help prevent further outbreaks, the pond should be drained, dried out, and disinfected with quicklime.

# ICHTHYOPHONUS

## SYSTEMATICS

The genus *Ichthyophonus*, as presently defined (Sprague, 1965), consists of two species: *I. hoferi* Plehn & Mulsow and *I. gasterophilum* (Caullery & Mesnil) Sprague. Little is known about *I. gasterophilum*. It was originally placed in the new genus *Ichthyosporidium* by Caullery & Mesnil (1905) who believed it to be congeneric with another organism described at the same time, *Ichthyosporidium phymogenes*. *I. gasterophilum* was found in the ducts of the gastric glands and in the pyloric caeca of two marine fishes, *Ciliata mustela* (= *Motella mustela*) and *Liparis liparis* (= *Liparis vulgaris*). *I. phymogenes* caused a tumour in the pectoral region of another marine fish, *Crenilabrus melops*. Caullery & Mesnil (1905) gave incomplete descriptions of these two new species and did not designate either one as a type species. It now appears that *I. gasterophilum* was possibly a fungus and *I. phymogenes* (now called *Ichthyosporidium giganteum* (Théolan) Swarczewsky 1914) was a protozoan. Thus over the years, the generic name *Ichthyosporidium* has been used by some authors to refer to organisms considered to be fungi (Pettit, 1911, 1913; Fish, 1934; Sproston, 1944; Sindermann & Scatterwood, 1954; Reichenbach-Klinke, 1954, 1955, 1960; Dorier & Degrange, 1961) whereas others used the name *Ichthyosporidium* to refer to a genus of protozoans.

In 1908, Robertson described a parasite of the flounder *Platichthys flesus* (= *Pleuronectes flesus*) which she thought was a protozoan, similar to *I. gasterophilum*, belonging in the genus *Ichthyosporidium*. Later, Plehn & Mulsow (1911) described a similar parasite from the rainbow trout (*Salmo gairdneri*) and, after studying the development of this organism in artificial culture media, they concluded that it was a fungus with chytridiaceous affinities. Plehn & Mulsow then went on to describe the monotypic fungal genus *Ichthyophonus* and called the single species *I. hoferi* in honour of Hofer who had noted what was thought to be the same disease in 1893 as the cause of a condition resulting in loss of equilibrium (Taumelkrankheit) in trout. Pettit (1911) believed that Robertson (1908) had studied a fungus and that this fungus was the same as the one studied by Plehn & Mulsow. Pettit (1913) transferred *Ichthyophonus hoferi* to the genus *Ichthyosporidium* and the new name for Plehn & Mulsow's organism became *Ichthyosporidium hoferi* (Plehn & Mulsow) Pettit. The name *Ichthyophonus hoferi* Plehn & Mulsow was rejected as a junior synonym. This change was not accepted by Neresheimer & Clodi (1914), Ellis (1928), Daniel (1933a,b), or Schäperclaus (1954) who preferred to retain the name *Ichthyophonus*. This latter viewpoint has been most recently supported by Sprague (1965) who made a convincing argument in favour of retaining the name *Ichthyophonus* for fungi and the name *Ichthyosporidium* for protozoans. Sprague (1966) went on to suggest that the name *Ichthyosporidium* may eventually be discarded as the presently recognized species in this genus are assigned to microsporidian genera.

Reichenbach-Klinke (1973) has suggested that *Ichthyophonus hoferi* might be identical with *I. gasterophilum* and that these species might also be identical to *Lymphosporidium truttae* described by Calkins (1900) as a parasite of *Salvelinus fontinalis*. The available data appear inadequate to give substance to these conjectures.

In addition to *I. hoferi* and *I. gasterophilum*, two other *Ichthyophonus* species have been described: *I. intestinalis* Léger & Hesse 1923 from *Salmo trutta* and other salmonids, and *I. lotae* Léger 1924 from *Lota lota* ( = *Lota vulgaris*). Both of these fungi were found only in the digestive tract and were believed not to be associated with any pathological condition. In a later paper, Léger (1927) reported that he had cultured "sphérules" presumed to be a stage in the developmental cycle of *I. intestinalis* and had found that these produced mycelia bearing asexual and sexual reproductive structures characteristic of the entomophthoracean genus *Basidiobolus*. Léger (1927) went on to suggest that *I. hoferi*, *I. intestinalis* and presumably *I. lotae* (although this was not specifically stated) should be transferred to the genus *Basidiobolus*. That is why the names *Basidiobolus intestinalis* (Léger & Hesse) Léger and

*B. lotae* (Léger) Léger occasionally appear in lists of species of fungi reported to be parasites of fishes.

From Léger's (1927) description and illustrations, it appears that his decision to transfer *I. intestinalis* to the genus *Basidiobolus* was quite reasonable. It was appparently accepted by Drechsler (1955); however, as Benjamin (1962) noted, the name *Basidiobolus intestinalis* was never validly published and the taxonomic status of both *B. intestinalis* and the very poorly described *B. lotae* will probably not be resolved satisfactorily since there are no extant cultures and the descriptions of these organisms are too inadequate to allow precise determinations. Proposals that *B. lotae* and *B. intestinalis* are the same organism (Reichenbach-Klinke, 1973) or that both species should be regarded as synonyms of *B. ranarum* (Ciferri, 1957) should, in our opinion, be dismissed as pure conjecture.

Subsequent to Léger's studies, *Basidiobolus ranarum* Eidam has been infrequently isolated from fishes (Nickerson & Hutchinson, 1971) and Yang (1962) has reported that *Basidiobolus meristosporus* Drechsler (a variety of *B. haptosporus* Drechsler fide Srinivasan & Thirumalachar, 1967) could infect young carp (*Cyprinus carpio*) and carp eggs; however, the evidence favouring the pathogenicity of *B. meristosporus* appears to be equivocal and, in our opinion, it remains to be proven whether a *Basidiobolus* species is capable of being an active fish pathogen.

Léger's (1927) decision to transfer *I. hoferi* to the genus *Basidiobolus* appears to have been based on two observations: first, he thought that the conidia produced in his cultures were similar to the structures found by Plehn & Mulsow (1911) in their cultures of *I. hoferi*; second, Léger concluded that the "sphérules" described by Pettit (1913) were similar to the "sphérules" of *I. intestinalis*. The first observation is of little value. The conidium illustrated by Léger (1927) bears a superficial resemblance to some of the structures illustrated by Plehn & Mulsow (1911) but the conclusion that the structures are homologous is not jutified. With regard to the second point, Dorier & Degrange (1961) concluded that the "sphérules" described by Pettit (1913) as a stage in the developmental cycle of *I. hoferi* were, in fact, a uninucleate stage of *Basidiobolus intestinalis*. One can only conclude that at our present level of understanding, there is little reason to suspect that *Basidiobolus* and *Ichthyophonus* will ever be shown to be congeneric.

Although there has been a general tendency to place the genus *Ichthyophonus* in the Entomophthorales, there is no definitive evidence favouring this viewpoint. Waterhouse (1973b) in a recent review of the taxonomy of the Entomophthorales, has excluded *Ichthyophonus* as a "doubtful genus." In our opinion, the evidence favouring the purported fungal affinities of *I. hoferi* is far from overwhelming and, as will be discussed in the following sections, resolution of these taxonomic problems is complicated by the fact that the name *I. hoferi* has probably been used to describe a complex of organisms and, as such, *I. hoferi* has become a "wastebasket" taxon with poorly defined species limits. Given the information presently available, and the absence of extant cultures of organisms thought to be *I. hoferi*, resolution of these problems is not possible.

## *ICHTHYOPHONUS HOFERI:* MORPHOLOGY AND DEVELOPMENT

There are five major publications relating morphology to developmental sequences in *I. hoferi*. Three of these studies (Daniel, 1933a; Fish, 1934; Sindermann & Scattergood, 1954) are primarily concerned with infections of Atlantic herring (*Clupea harengus harengus*) in the western North Atlantic and one study (Sproston, 1944) is concerned with infections of Atlantic mackerel (*Scomber scombrus*) in the eastern North Atlantic. These four studies have been very adequately summarized by Johnson & Sparrow (1961). The most recent study (Dorier & Degrange, 1961) is concerned with infections of freshwater salmonids (*Salmo gairdneri, Salvelinus fontinalis*) in Europe. Dorier & Degrange (1961) also provided a critical summary of the pertinent aspects of the study by Neresheimer & Clodi (1914), who also investigated the development of *Ichthyophonus* infections in European salmonids.

*I. hoferi* most frequently occurs in the tissues of infected fish as a spherical, thick-walled, multinucleate cell (Figs. 10, 11; Plates 20, 21, 23) variously called a "cyst," "spore," "resting stage" or

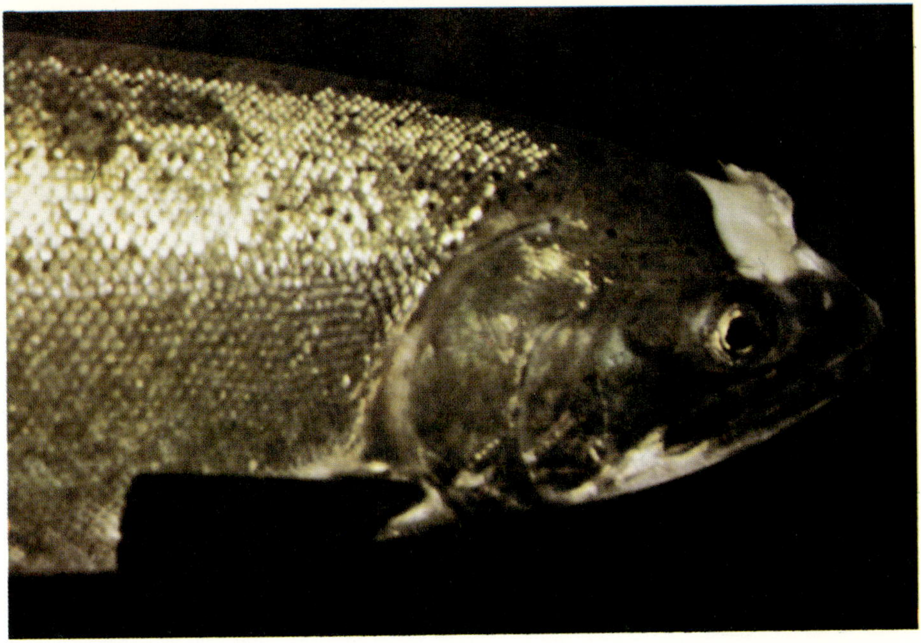

Plate 1. Coho salmon *(Oncorhynchus kisutch)* with saprolegniosis. The apparent initial site of infection is a trauma on the dorsal surface of the head.

Plate 2. Moribund chinook salmon *(Oncorhynchus tshawytscha)* with severe saprolegniosis.

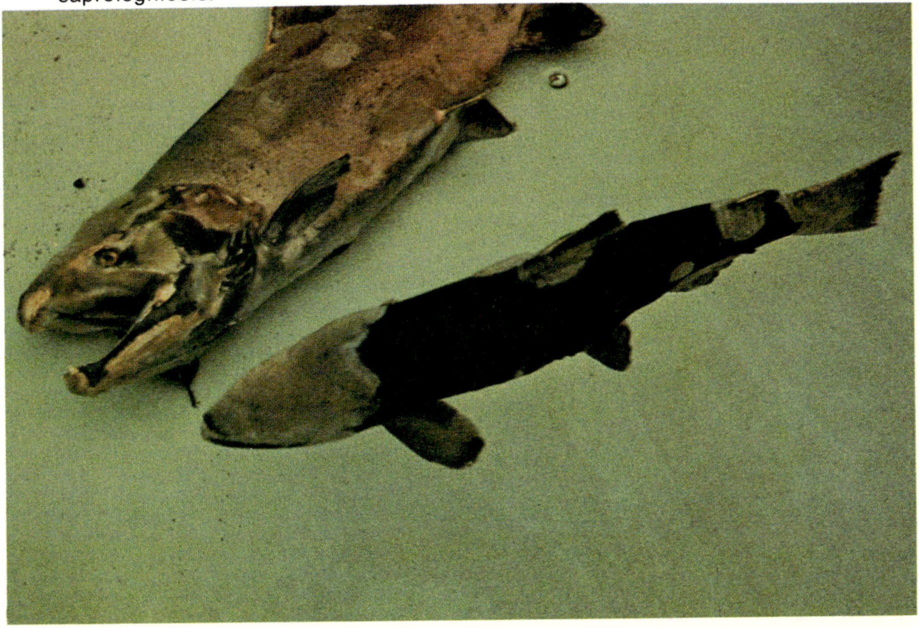

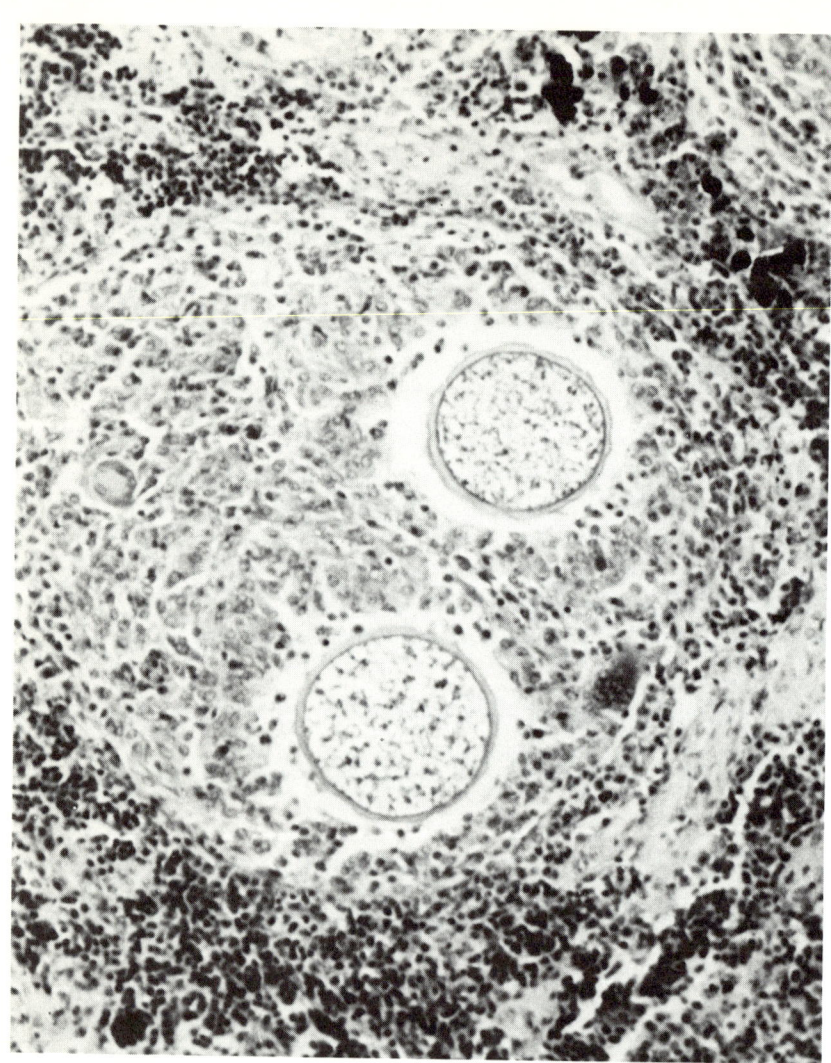

Fig. 10. *Ichthyophonus hoferi*. Resting spores eliciting a severe granulomatous response and giant cells in spleen of fish. X 160, H & E. (Photograph courtesy of R. E. Wolke, from "Pathology of Bacterial and Fungal Diseases Affecting Fish," in William E. Ribelin & George Migaki, eds., *The Pathology of Fishes* (Madison: The University of Wisconsin Press; Copyright 1975 by the Board of Regents of the University of Wisconsin System), pp. 94-97.)

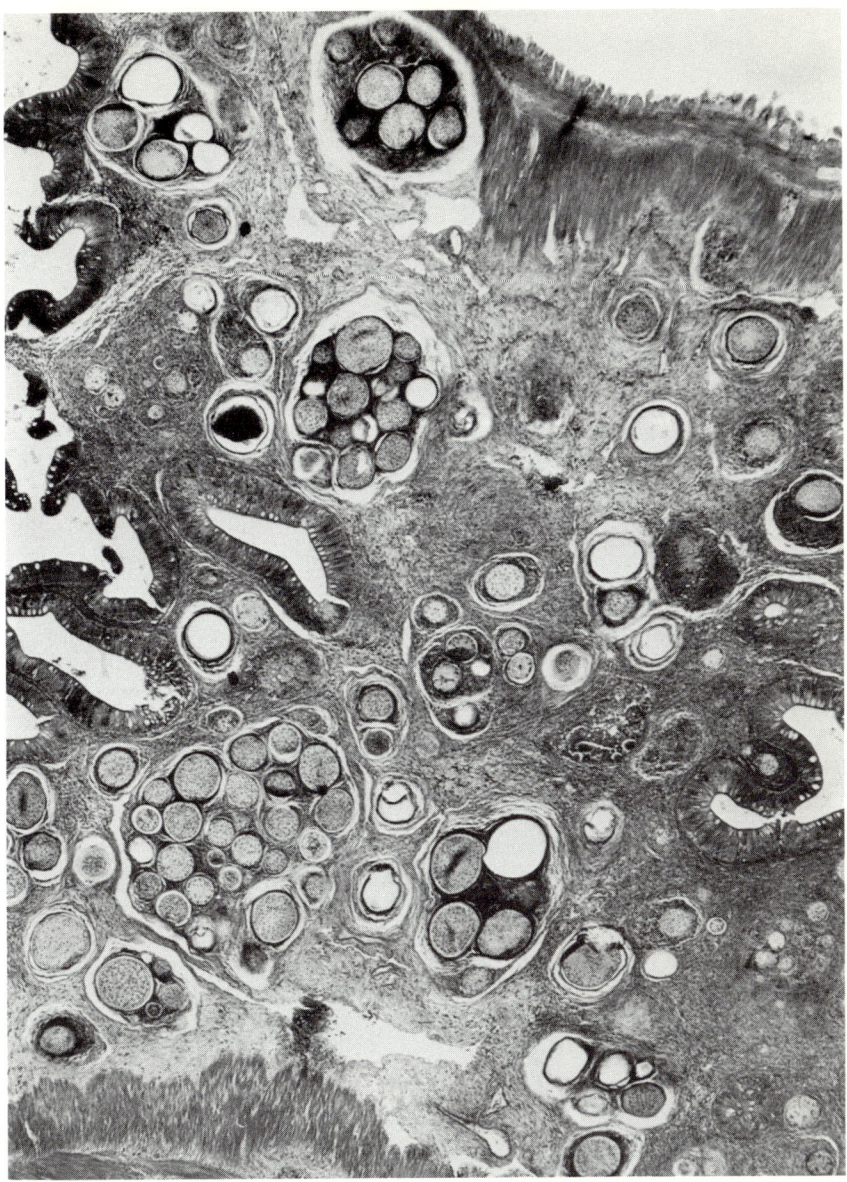

Fig. 11. *Ichthyophonus* resting spores in the intestine of the yellowtail flounder (*Limanda ferruginea*). (Photograph courtesy of Geo. D. Ruggieri and R.F. Nigrelli.)

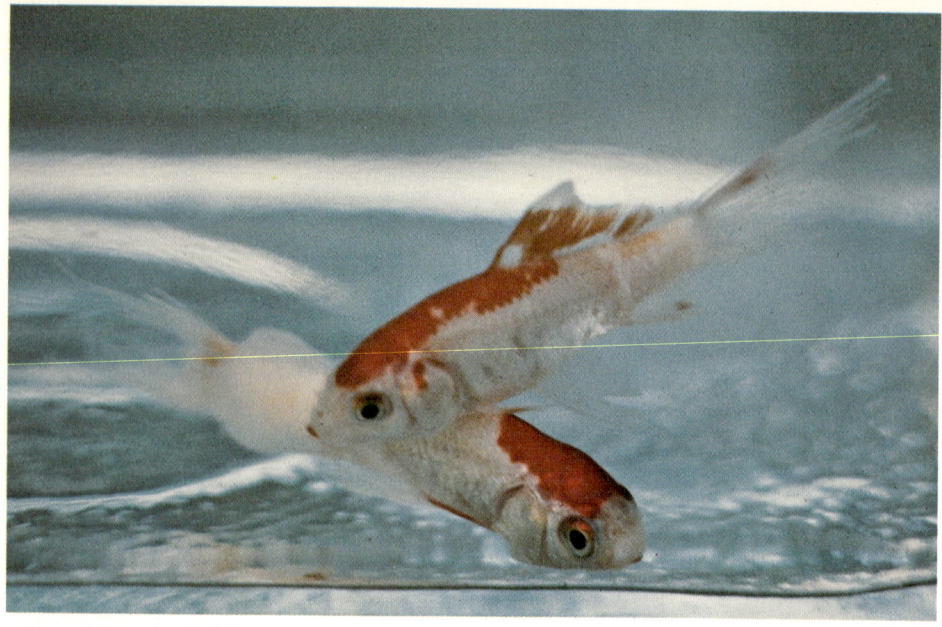

Plate 3. Goldfish (*Carassius auratus*) with *Saprolegnia* infections in the region of their caudal peduncles.
Plate 4. Caudal peduncle of a guppy *(Poecilia reticulata)* shown 24 hours after it was wounded and inoculated with a *Saprolegnia* isolate. (Photograph courtesy of N. Nolard-Tintigner, with permission of Acta Zoologica et Pathologica Antverpiensia.)

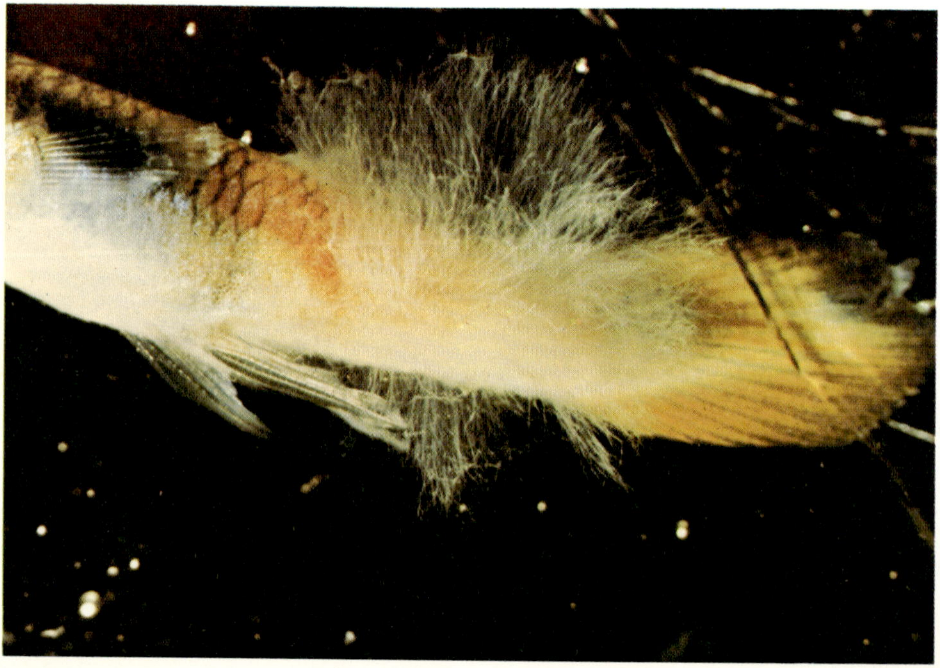

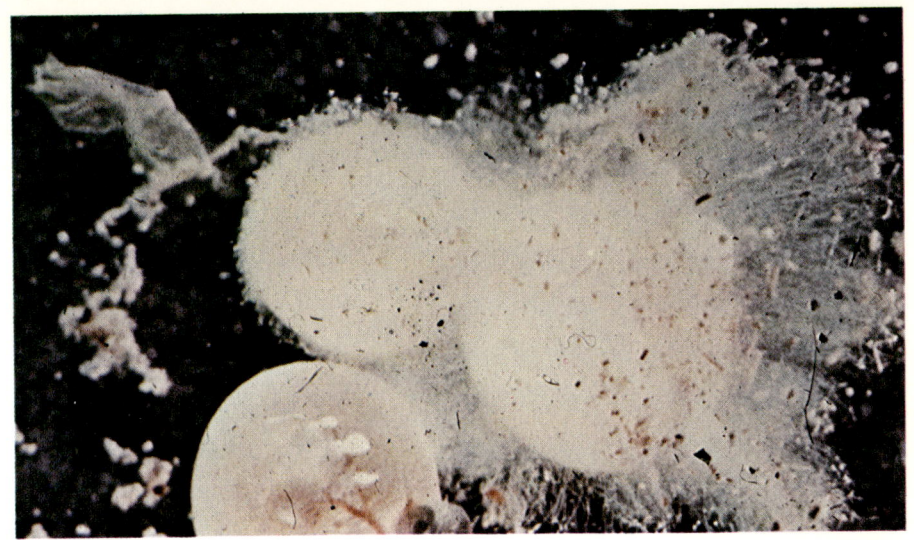

Plate 5. Saprolegniosis of rainbow trout *(Salmo gairdneri)* eggs. (Photograph courtesy of H.-H. Reichenbach-Klinke).

Plate 6, 7. Comparison of uninfected (Plate 6) and infected (Plate 7) skin and muscle tissue from a sockeye salmon (*Oncorhynchus nerka*). Note the loss of epidermis and scales and the penetration of the hyphae through the *stratum compactum* of the dermis into the hypodermis and musculature. PAS-light green; X 70.

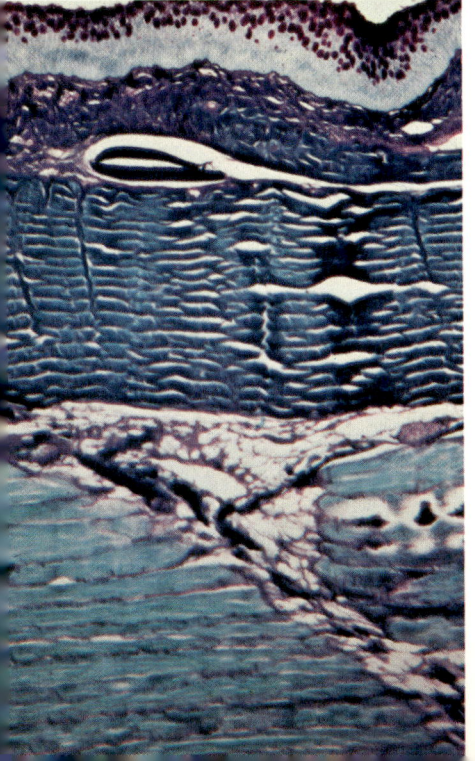
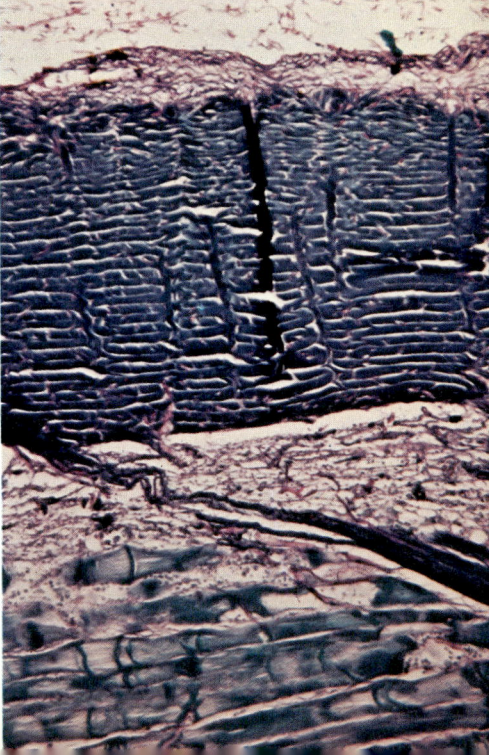

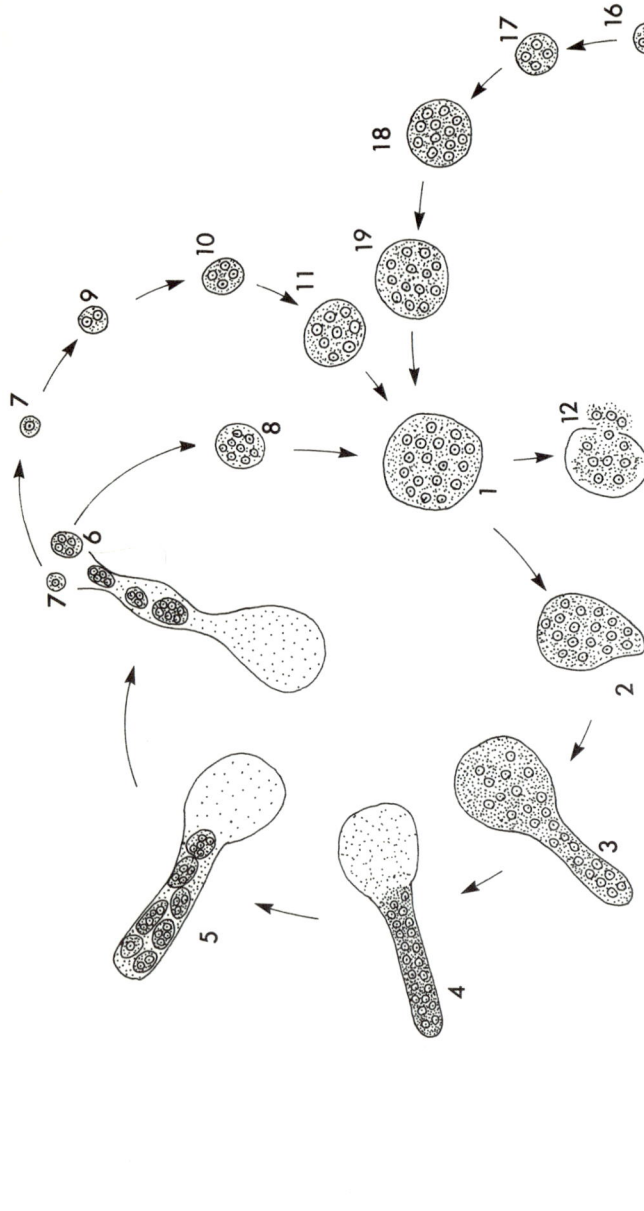

Fig. 12. Developmental cycle of *Ichthyophonus hoferi* according to Daniel (1933a), showing development of a stout hypha and formation of "daughter spores" (Stages 1-5), development of a resting spore from a daughter spore (Stages 7-11), and development of a resting spore by "fragmentation" (Stages 12-19).

"resting spore." The use of the word "cyst" is clearly inappropriate in this context. This term should more properly refer to the capsule of connective tissue and reticulo-endothelial cells which *encyst* the parasite, with a number of cysts composing a *nodule* (Robertson, 1909). We shall generally use the term "resting spore" in later sections of this chapter while at the same time acknowledging that this term implies that the cell is metabolically inactive, an assumption which may not be justified. In the following discussion of development and morphology, we adopt the terminology employed by the original investigators to describe their material, rather than attempt to adopt a standardized terminology for structures which may not be homologous.

The resting spores vary in size between 10-250 microns in diameter. The nuclei have a diameter of roughly 2-4 microns and various authors have noted that it contains a prominent centrally located karyosome with fine "rays" connecting it to granules associated with the nuclear membrane. The chromatin appears to be arranged in a ring around the periphery of the karyosome (Dorier & Degrange, 1961). The cytoplasm gives a positive PAS and Bauer reaction which indicates that it contains glycogen, a common reserve carbohydrate in fungi. The wall of the resting spore gives a strong PAS reaction which indicates that it's composed of polysaccharides as, indeed, it would have to be if we are going to entertain the notion that *I. hoferi* is a fungus. The wall of the resting spore has a variable thickness (approximately 2-11 microns) and, according to Amlacher (1965), may consist of as many as three layers.

Both Daniel (1933a) and Fish (1934) agree that the resting spore in herring can germinate to produce a multinucleate stout hypha. According to Daniel, the cytoplasm then evacuates the spore into the hypha and this is followed by endogenous cleavage to produce "daughter spores" of varying sizes and numbers of nuclei (Fig. 12). Alternatively, the resting spore may produce "daughter spores" endogenously without prior formation of a hypha. Fish (1934) agrees with these two basic patterns, but does not describe or illustrate the cytoplasmic evacuation of the resting spore prior to "daughter spore" cleavage. Fish also noted that the hypha could branch, although not extensively. Both Daniel and Fish agree that the "daughter spores," subsequent to cleavage, are

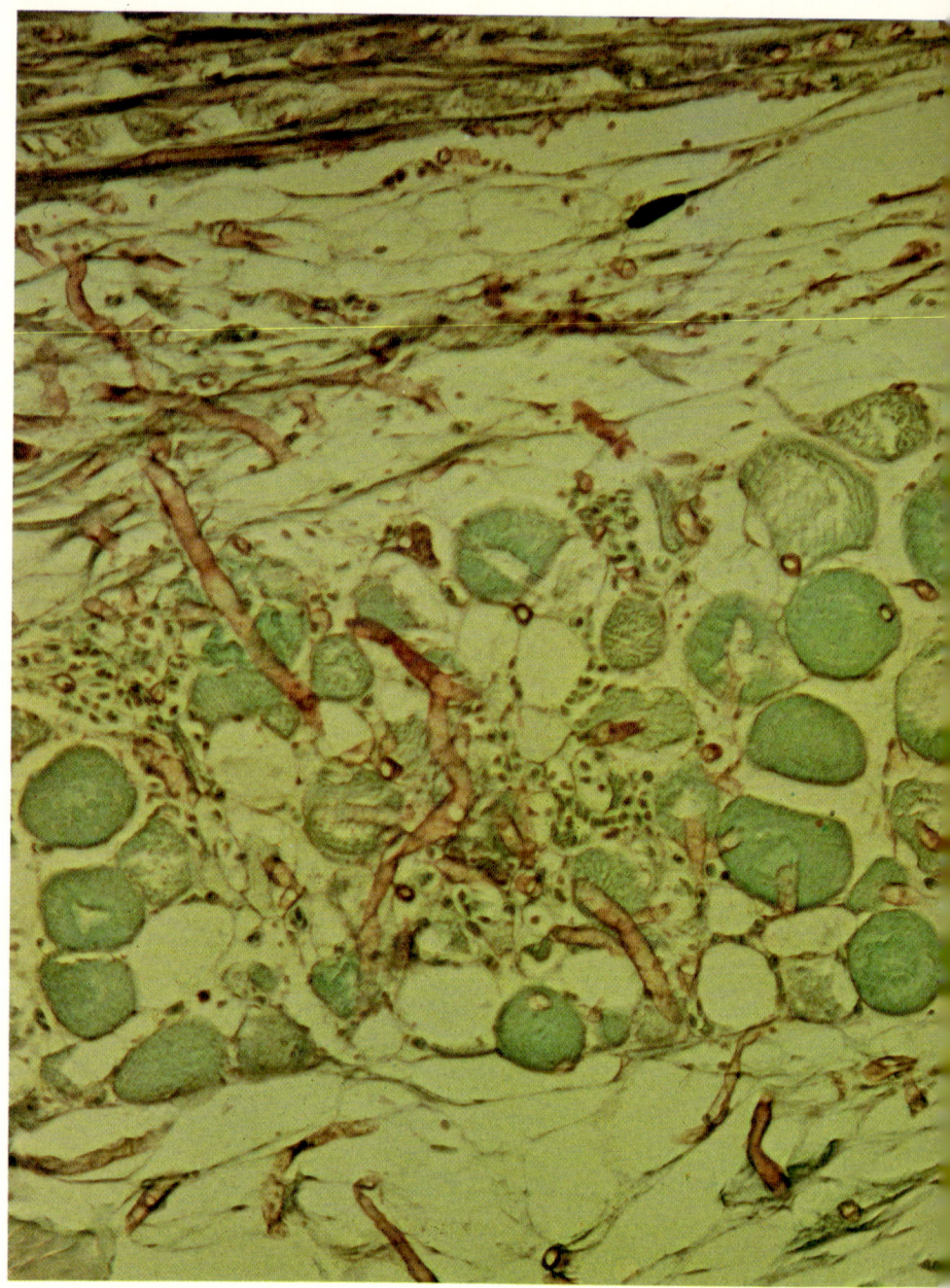

Plate 8. Infected sockeye salmon (*Oncorhynchus nerka*) tissue at a higher magnification showing saprolegnian hyphae (pink-red strands) in the hypodermis and musculature. PAS-light green; X 260.

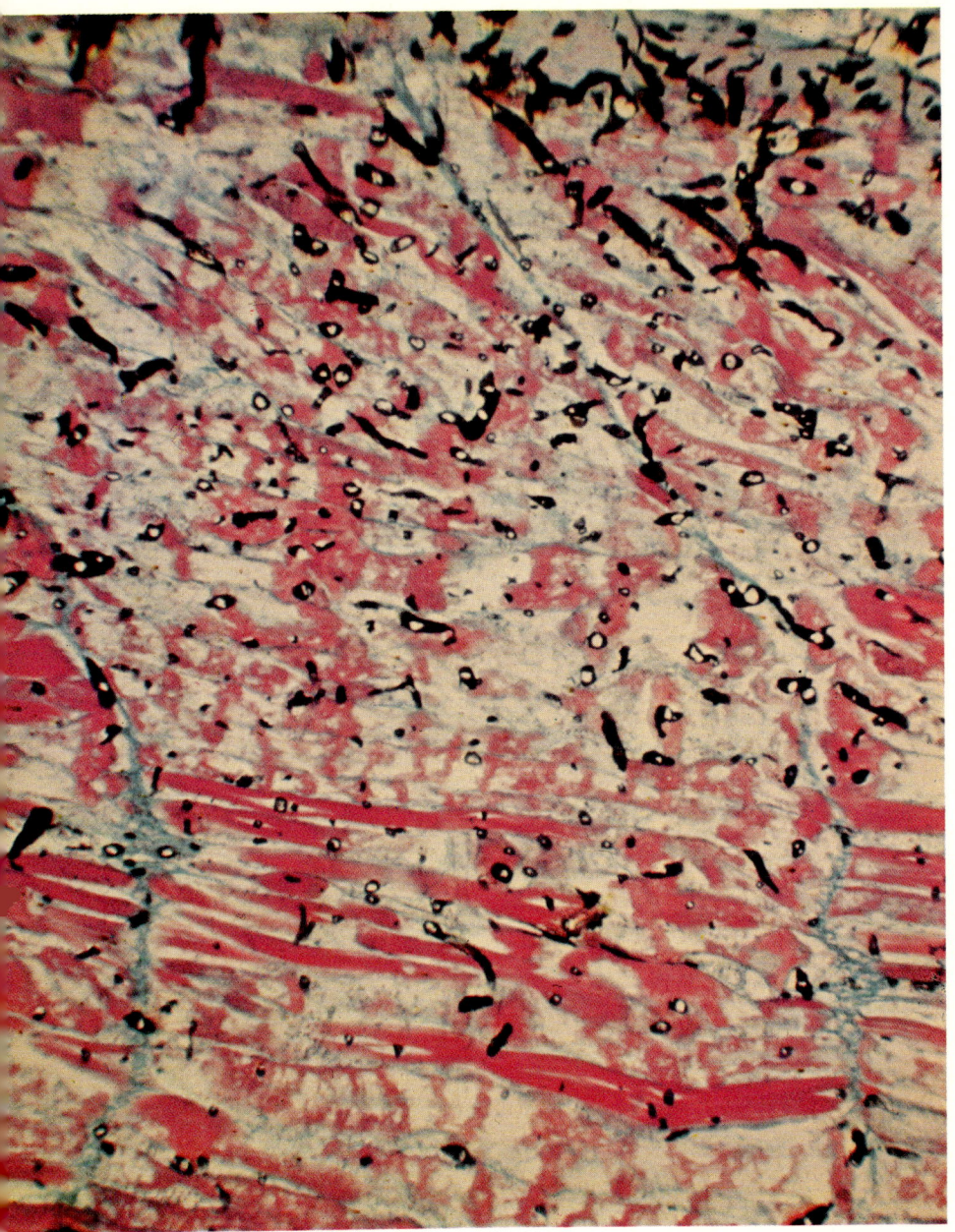

Plate 9. Muscle tissue from a guppy (*Poecilia reticulata*) experimentally infected by *Achlya* sp. In this case the tissue was stained by the Gomori-Grocott methenamine silver technique which stains the hyphae brown-black. Note the similarity of this material to Plates 7 and 8, particularly with regard to the necrosis of the muscle tissue and the apparent absence of an inflammatory response. (Photograph courtesy of N. Nolard-Tintigner.)

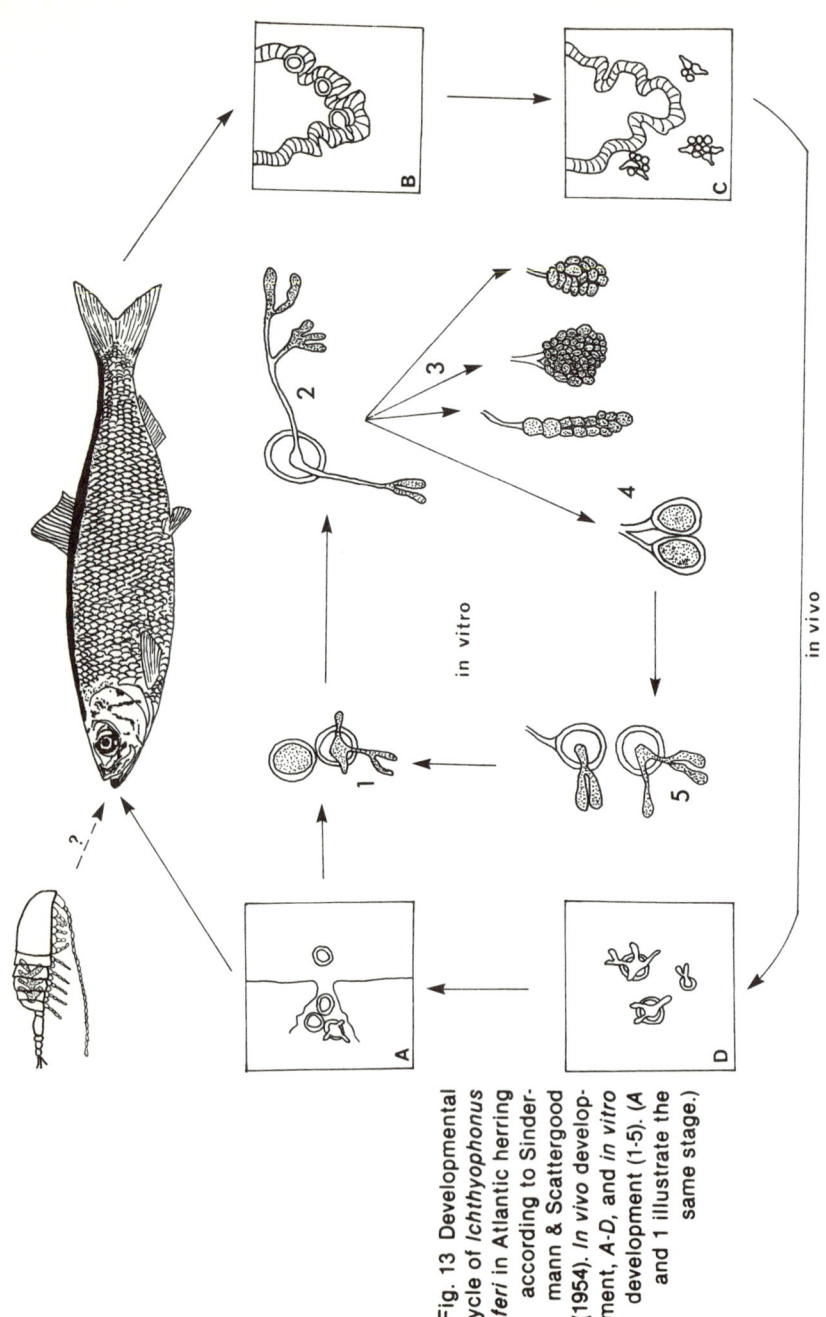

Fig. 13 Developmental cycle of *Ichthyophonus hoferi* in Atlantic herring according to Sindermann & Scattergood (1954). *In vivo* development, A-D, and *in vitro* development (1-5). (A and 1 illustrate the same stage.)

released by rupture of the hypha or, if no hypha is produced, by the rupture of the resting spore wall.

In addition to the "daughter spore" formation, Daniel (1933a) tentatively suggested that there might be a third developmental pattern which he called "fragmentation." In this pattern, the wall of the resting spore ruptures and releases the nuclei each of which "... is surrounded by minute bits of cytoplasm" and subsequently these become enclosed by a wall and develop into the multinucleate resting spores (Fig. 12). Fish (1934) did not agree with this observation and maintained that although normal nuclei and cytoplasm could be observed "... scattered through the tissues," close examination revealed that they were always enclosed by a hyphal wall which was "... easily overlooked because of its transparency."

The developmental pattern described by Sindermann & Scattergood (1954) for what is presumably the same organism (Fig. 13) differs somewhat from the pattern described by Daniel (1933a) and Fish (1934). According to Sindermann & Scattergood, the resting spore produces multiple germ tubes and these, *in vivo*, are blunt pseudopodium-like hyphae which extend for a maximum length of 3-4 times the diameter of the resting spore. This is in marked contrast to the results reported by Fish (1934) who noted that only a single germ tube was produced and that the hypha could attain a maximum length of 20-25 times the diameter of the resting spore. Following germination, according to Sindermann & Scattergood, the cytoplasm evacuates the resting spore (presumably in a manner analogous to that described by Daniel, 1933a) and this is followed by endogenous cleavage to produce from five to several hundred aplanetic propagules which Sindermann & Scattergood call "hyphal bodies." The "hyphal bodies" can subsequently grow into new spores. As Johnson & Sparrow (1961) have noted, it appears that the "hyphal bodies" of Sindermann & Scattergood can be produced in much greater numbers than the "daughter spores" described by Daniel (1933a) and Fish (1934), so it is hard to know if these authors were describing the same phenomenon. Sindermann & Scattergood also noted that endogenous cleavage could occur in the resting spore without prior hyphal development.

Sindermann & Scattergood (1954) also studied *in vitro* develop-

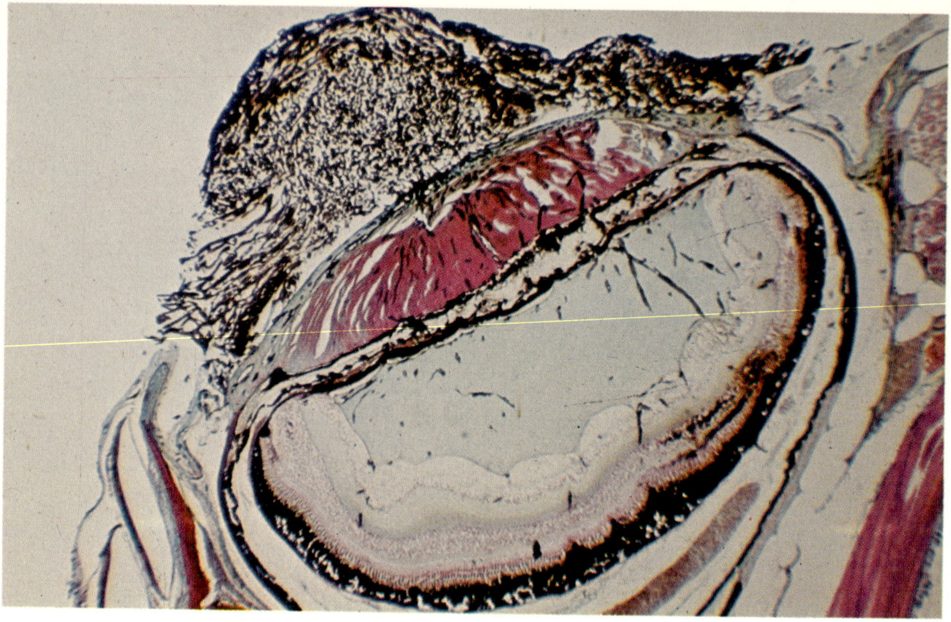

Plate 10. Eye of a guppy *(Poecilia reticulata)* infected by *Achyla klebsiana*. Gomori-Grocott. (Photograph courtesy of N. Nolard-Tintigner.)

Plate 11. Spinal cord of a swordtail *(Xiphophorus helleri)* experimentally infected by a *Saprolegnia* isolate. Gomori-Grocott. (Photograph courtesy of N. Nolard Tintigner, with permission of Acta Zoologica et Pathologica Antverpiensia.)

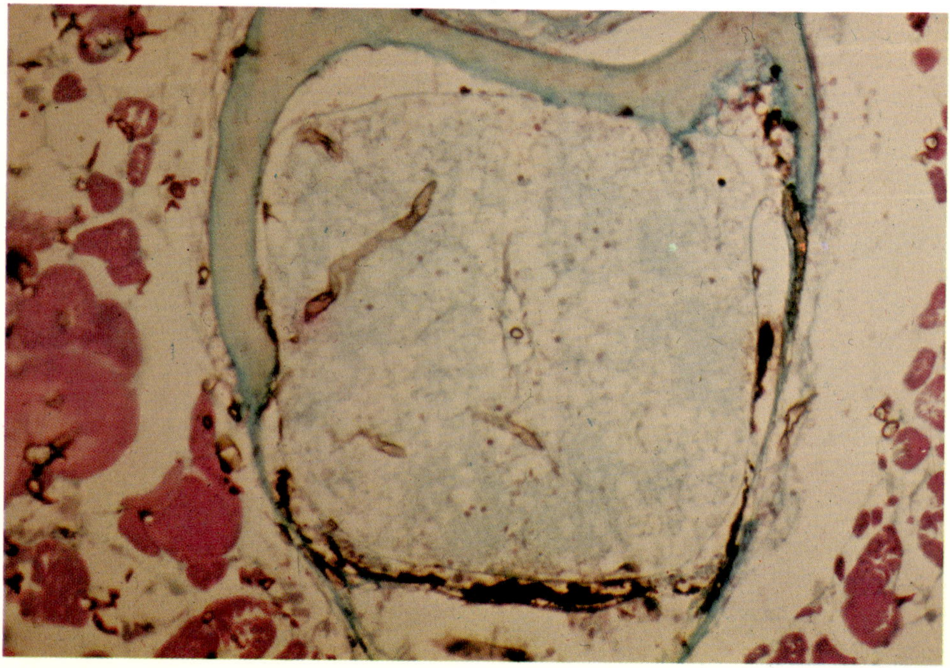

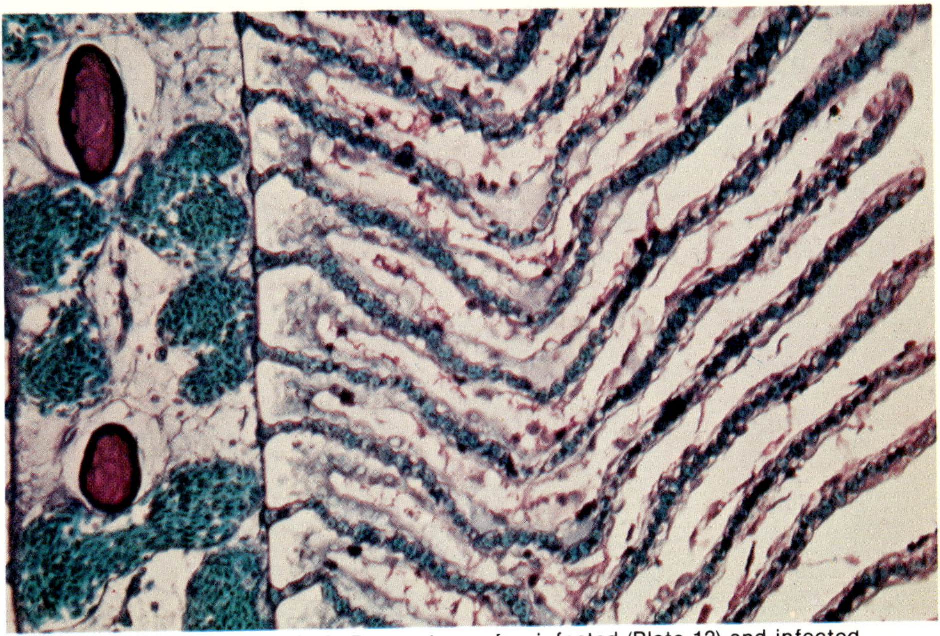

Plates 12 (above) and 13. Comparison of uninfected (Plate 12) and infected (Plate 13) gill lamellae from an adult male coho salmon *(Oncorhynchus kisutch)*. The two deep purplish red areas on the left in Plate 12 are cartilage in the gill filament; the strong greenish blue areas are masses of erythrocytes. In Plate 13 the pink areas on the right and in the center are saprolegnian hyphae. PAS-light green; X 73.

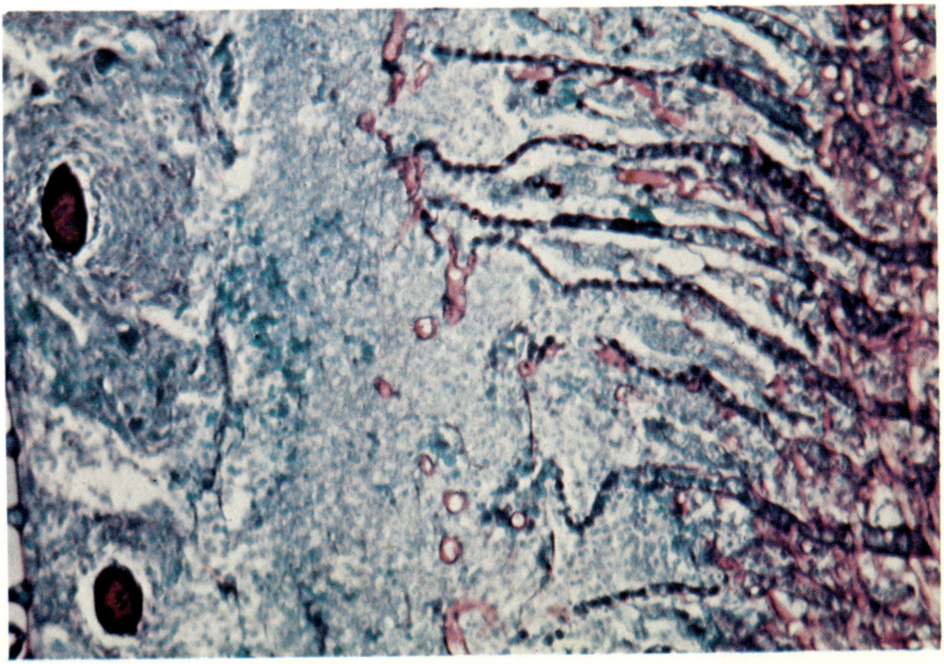

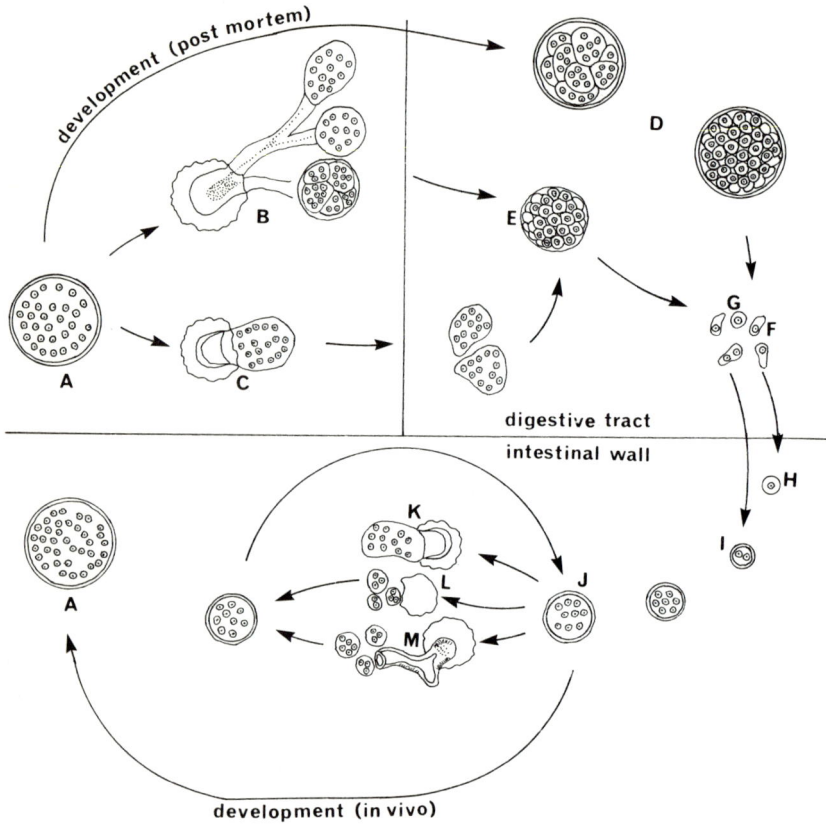

Fig. 14. Developmental cycle of *Ichthyophonus hoferi* in freshwater salmonids according to Dorier & Degrange (1961). See text for explanation.

ment of *I. hoferi* (Fig. 13). Other authors (Plehn & Mulsow, 1911; Fish, 1934; Forster, 1941; Reichenbach-Klinke, 1954, 1960; see Plate 22) have reported the successful culture of *I. hoferi*, but Sindermann & Scattergood's study appears to be the one that describes its cultural characteristics in most detail.

The inoculum that Sindermann & Scattergood used for this work consisted of fungal material removed aseptically from the heart or lateral musculature of the herring. This material was inoculated directly into the surface of agar slants of Sabouraud's dextrose medium[1] supplemented by 1% beef serum. Usually germination and growth from the inoculum was noted 7-10 days after inoculation. Growth could occur within a range of 3-20°C with the apparent optimum being 10°C. Only the large "quiescent spores" germinated and they produced long, slender, branching coenocytic hyphae with bulbous tips. The hyphae developed principally beneath the surface of the agar and were much more extensive than the hyphae observed in the fish. When the cultures reached a diameter of 5-15 mm after 30-60 days, growth virtually stopped, but cultures could remain viable for at least as long as fourteen months.

The cytoplasm evacuated the spore almost immediately after germination and became concentrated near the advancing hyphal tip, where it was eventually cleaved either into numerous "hyphal bodies" which did not germinate in culture or into heavy-walled spores which would occasionally germinate in culture (Fig. 13).

According to Dorier & Degrange (1961), the developmental cycle of *I. hoferi* in infected freshwater salmonids in Europe can be summarized as follows:

The fish are infected by ingestion of latent "cysts" (resting spores) (Fig. 14A). Some of these "cysts" are transformed directly into "amoebablasts" and undergo endogenous cytoplasmic cleavage (Fig. 14D). Other "cysts" germinate by producing a filament or hyphae (Fig. 14B) or by releasing a "plasmodium" (Fig.

---

[1] The exact composition of this medium was not given by Sindermann & Scattergood. It can consist of 1-1.5% peptone, 2.0% glucose or maltose and 1.25-3.5% agar. 0.5% glycerine is also added sometimes. Various variants of this medium, with appropriate antibiotics added to it, are frequently used for the isolation of pathogenic fungi (Conant et. al., 1971; Stevens, 1974).

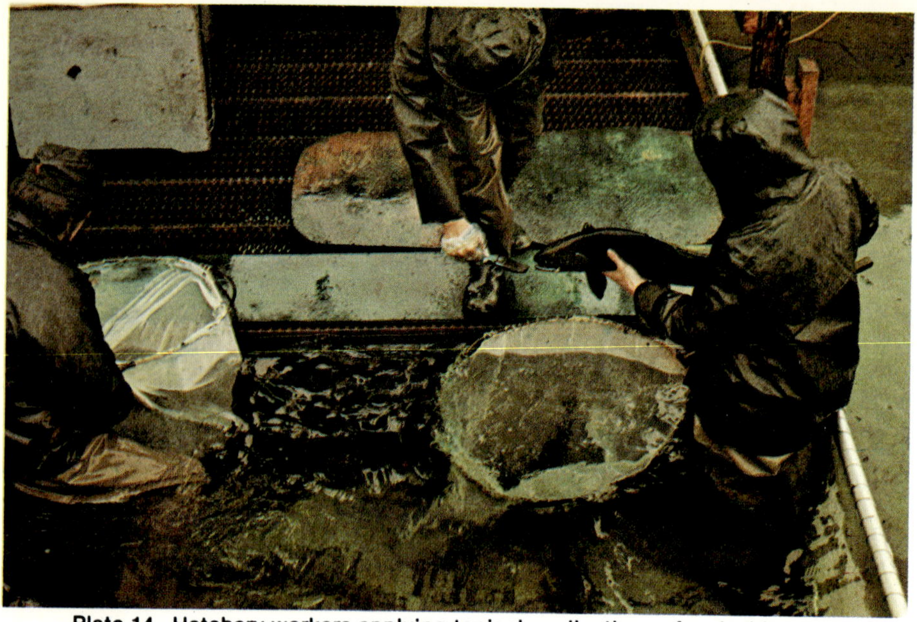

Plate 14. Hatchery workers applying topical applications of malachite green to Pacific salmon with saprolegniasis.

Plate 15. Carp (*Cyprinus carpio*) with operculum removed to show the gross appearance of branchiomycosis. (Photograph by courtesy of Dr. H.-H. Reichenbach-Klinke.)

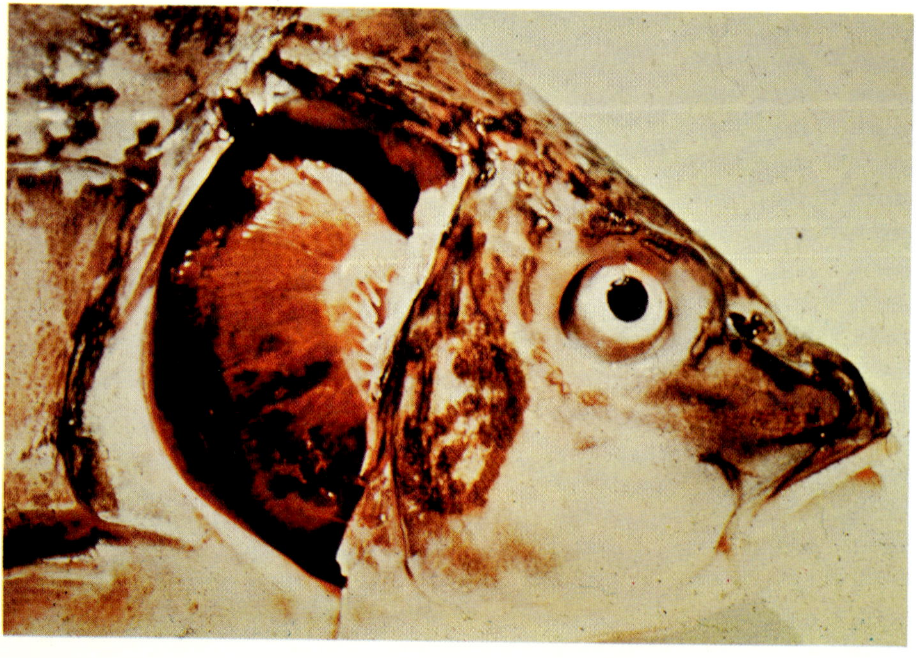

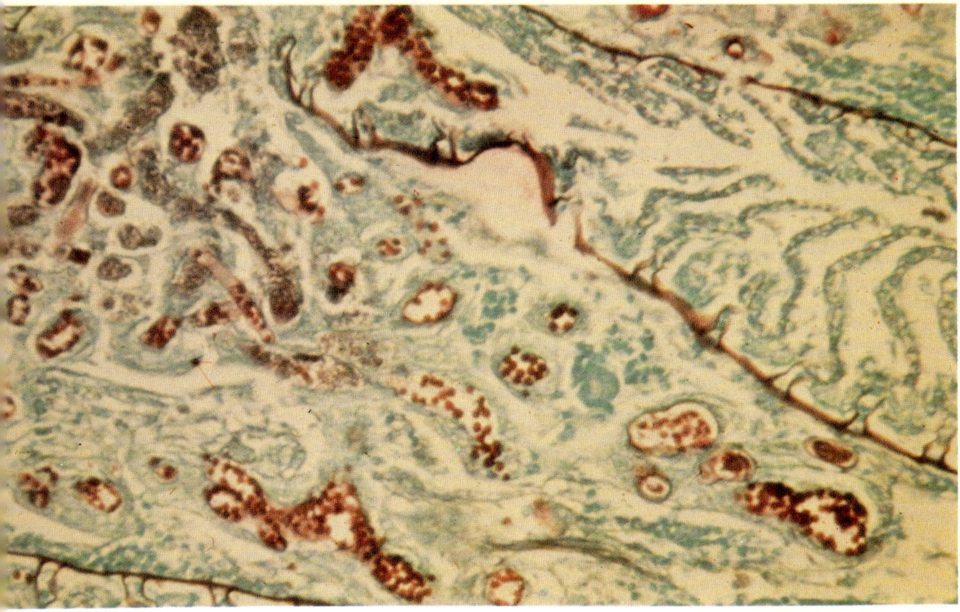

Plate 16. *Branchiomyces* sp. in the gills of a carp (*Cyprinus carpio*). (Photograph courtesy of R.J. Roberts.)

Plate 17. *Branchiomyces* sp. from the gills of a bleak (*Alburnus alburnus alborella*) from Lago Maggiore, Italy. Squash mount in polyvinyl lactophenol blue; X 370. (Photograph courtesy of R. Peduzzi.)

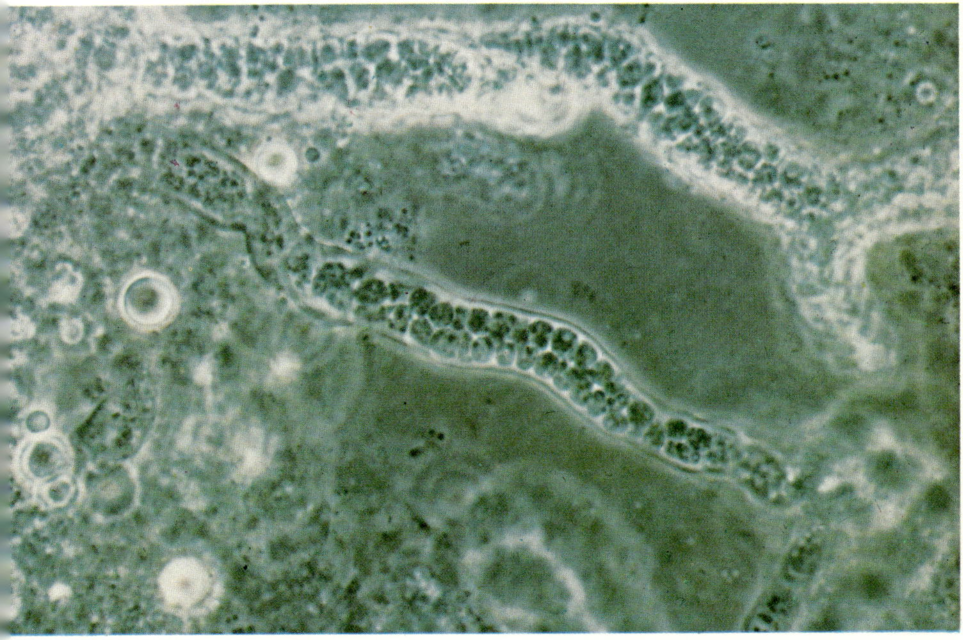

14C). These latter two methods of germination result in the production of "amoebablasts" with thinner walls and a smaller size than the others (Fig. 14E).

The walls of the "amoebablasts" rupture and typically uni- or binucleate "amoeboid forms" are released into the intestine. Some of these "amoeboid forms" do not develop further but become inactive and assume a spherical shape (Fig. 14H). When voided with the faeces they are destroyed by direct contact with the water. Other "amoeboid forms" succeed in penetrating the wall of the intestine and they are transported in the blood to the viscera or musculature where they turn into uni- or binucleate "cysts" (Fig. 14I). These "cysts" grow rapidly, become multinucleate, accumulate reserves of lipid and glycogen, and turn into "latent cysts" which become encapsulated by the host (Fig. 14A). Other "cysts" may release a "plasmodium" (Fig. 14K) or produce "spores" by endogenous cleavage which are subsequently released either by rupture of the "cyst" wall (Fig. 14L) or through the ends of a short, irregular and striated hypha (Fig. 14M). These "endospores" or "plasmodia" can initiate secondary infection of the host.

*Ichthyophonus hoferi* in mackerel, as described by Sproston (1944), exhibits a high degree of polymorphism which includes the following structures: (1) large elongated "chlamydospores" with a hard exospore; (2) "dome-shaped conidia" thought to be similar to those produced by entomophthoracean fungi; (3) "hyphal bodies" (not to be confused with the "hyphal bodies" described by Sindermann & Scattergood, 1954) of varying shape which can round up and become encysted; (4) "branched conidiophores" containing "endo-conidia" which are liberated as amoeboid bodies into the blood vessels; (5) "simple clavate sporangia" which also contain "endo-conidia"; (6) "hyphal fusions" which can proceed to further outgrowths of similar hyphae; and finally, (7) "spores produced by hyphal fusion" which are described as "resting spores" with a thick resistant wall and which were thought to be the means of dispersal to new suscepts. These structures and their proposed relationship to one another are shown in Figure 44 of Sproston's paper.

If we assume that all the developmental stages described by Sproston (1944) do, in fact, belong to the same organism, then it appears unlikely that it is the same as *I. hoferi* sensu Sindermann & Scattergood or *I. hoferi* sensu Dorier & Degrange. Sproston's results have not been corroborated and, except for the summary by Johnson & Sparrow (1961), recent authors (Reichenbach-Klinke & Elkan, 1965; Amlacher, 1970; Sindermann, 1970; van Duijn, 1973; Reichenbach-Klinke, 1973; Wolke, 1975; Alderman, 1976) have either completely ignored Sproston's work or have only accorded it superficial and cursory treatment. Sproston (1944) attempted to reconcile her results with those of previous investigators, and Johnson & Sparrow (1961) attempted to reconcile Sproston's observations with Sindermann & Scattergood's (1954) results; nevertheless, Sproston's *I. hoferi* remains an enigmatic organism.

Further morphological variations have been attributed to *I. hoferi* by Reichenbach-Klinke (1954, 1956a,b, 1973) and Reichenbach-Klinke & Elkan (1965) who reported that the "plasmodium" can produce broad, tubular, club-shaped "macrohyphae" (7-15 microns wide) or slender non-septate filaments 2-3 microns wide called "microhyphae." Chains of brown, thick-walled "endoconidia" about 1.5-4.0 microns in diameter may be constricted from the ends of the "microhyphae" but can apparently also be produced without any hyphal development. According to Reichenbach-Klinke, "microhyphae" are found only in marine fish. Other types of spores found in marine fish include "conidia" 10-20 microns wide, and putative "resting spores" 4-6 microns wide. In tropical freshwater fishes, the development of the "macrohyphae" may be very restricted with divisions into "daughter plasmodia" occurring immediately after germination. In culture (Reichenbach-Klinke, 1954), a structure called a "knee cell" (incorrectly translated as an ascus in Reichenbach-Klinke, 1973) was produced. The significance of this finding is not known.

Schäperclaus (1953), Reichenbach-Klinke (1956c), and Reichenbach-Klinke & Elkan (1965) have discussed the possibility that there may be two species or forms of *Ichthyophonus*. The first form, known as the "salmonid form," would occur in freshwater and marine fish from cold-water environments and, briefly, would be characterized by the ability to produce long, germinative tubular hyphae and by the absence of pigmentation of the "cysts."

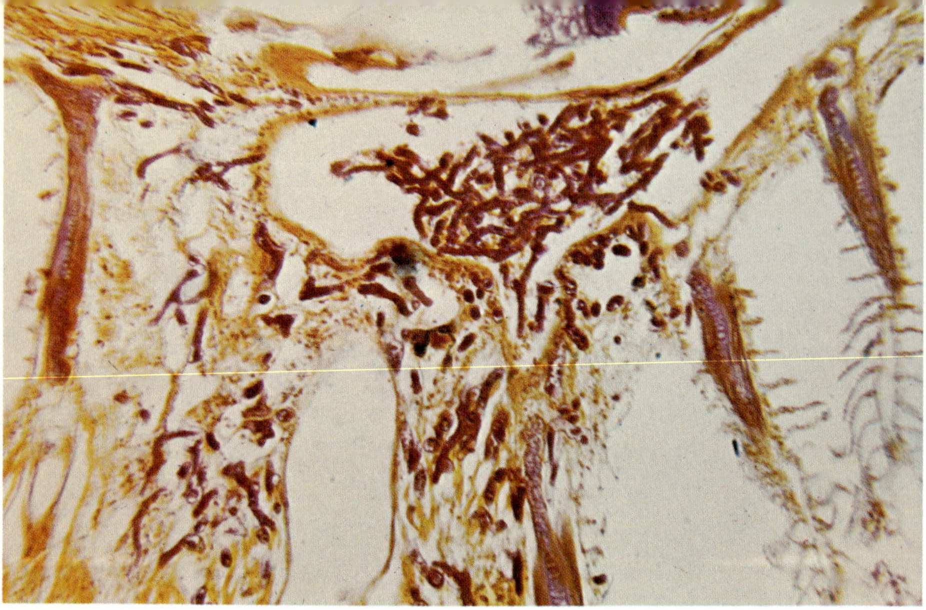

Plate 18 (above). Hyphae of *Branchiomyces* sp. in the gills of a bleak *(Alburnus alburnus alborella)* from Lake Maggiore, Italy. Gridley; X 45. (Photograph courtesy of G. Giussani, I. Boroni and E. Grimaldi with permission of the Memorie dell' Instituto Italiano Idrobiologia.) Plate 19 (below). Trout with an *Ichthyophonus* infection of the brain. Note the spinal curvature. (Photograph courtesy of the Western Fish Disease Laboratory, Seattle, Washington.)

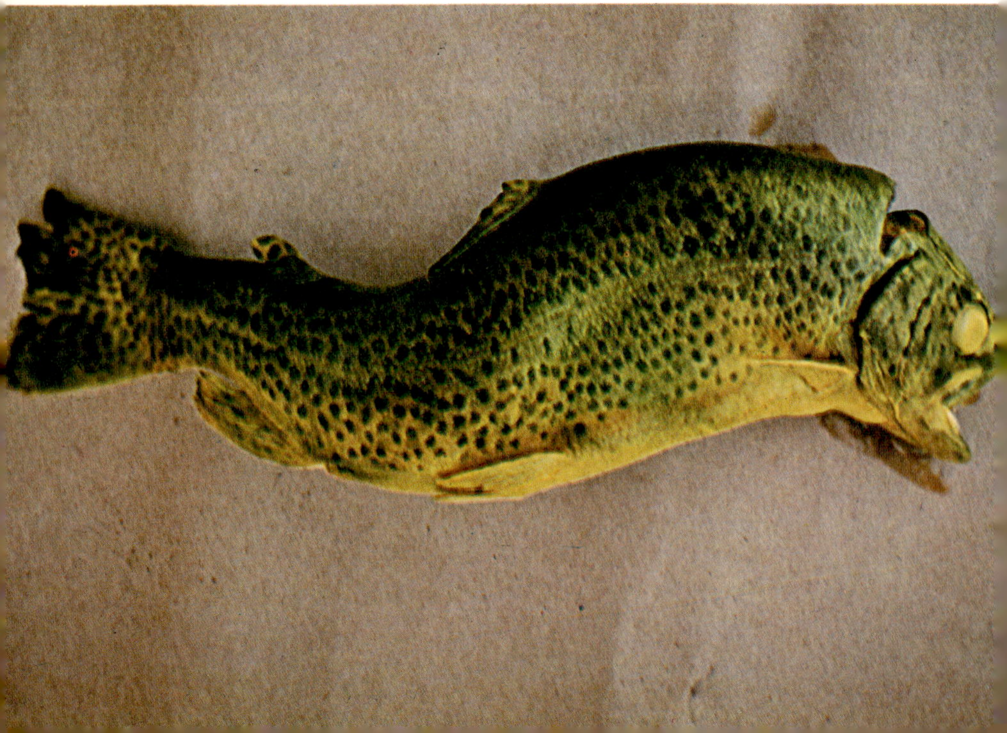

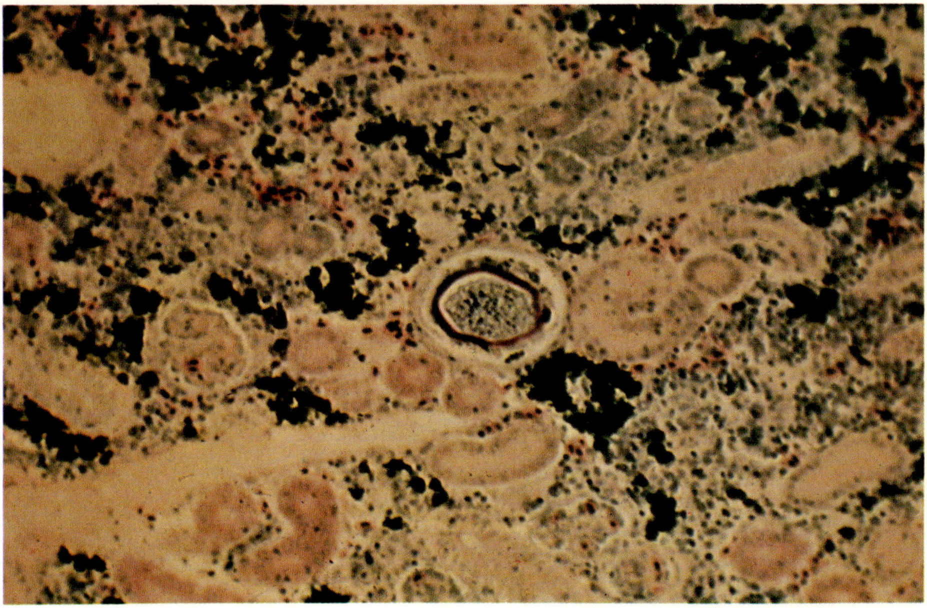

Plate 20. *Ichthyophonus* "resting spore" in the kidney of a rainbow trout (*Salmo gairdneri*). May-Gruenwald Giemsa. (Photograph by courtesy of the Western Fish Disease Laboratory, Seattle, Washington.)

Plate 21. *Ichthyophonus* "resting spores" in the brain of a rainbow trout (*Salmo gairdneri*). May-Gruenwald Giemsa. (Photograph by courtesy of the Western Fish Disease Laboratory, Seattle, Washington.)

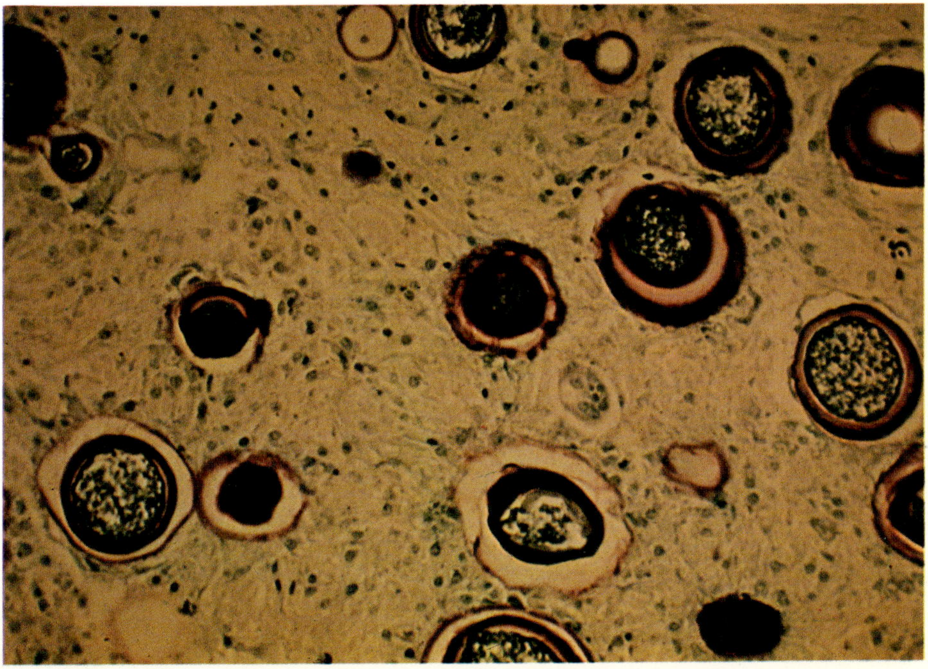

The second form, called the "aquarium fish form," would generally be found in freshwater tropical fish and would be characterized by the general absence of hyphae and by the presence of degenerate, heavily melanized "cysts." Later Reichenbach-Klinke (1973) concluded, on the basis of cultures obtained from a *Symphysodon* species (Plate 22) and from infection experiments carried out by H. Herkner (1961), that both forms belonged to the same species.

It appears that much of the supposed polymorphism attributed to *I. hoferi* may be related to problems in distinguishing among *Ichthyophonus* infections and infections caused by other organisms which also elicit a chronic, proliferative, granulomatous response. This problem of differential diagnosis has been briefly discussed by Meuron & Burgisser (1973) and by Wolke (1975). The most extensive study to date, however, is the detailed investigation by Amlacher (1965). Amlacher studied *Ichthyophonus* infections by rainbow trout and a variety of freshwater aquarium fish with putative *Ichthyophonus* infections. Based on histopathological studies, culture studies, and infection experiments, Amlacher concluded that the "aquarium fish" *Ichthyophonus* infections actually represented symptoms of piscine tuberculosis caused by acid-fast bacteria. While more research should be done in this area, it appears that the prudent investigator should, at the very least, stain material suspected to be an *Ichthyophonus* infection by the Ziehl-Neelson method for acid-fast bacteria, especially when involved with freshwater tropical fish.

## *ICHTHYOPHONUS HOFERI*: PATHOLOGY AND EPIZOOTIOLOGY

In the following discussion we are adopting the position that the major studies concerned with *Ichthyophonus* infections of fishes from the North Atlantic (Table VI) and of salmonids from Europe and North America (Table VII) may not be concerned with the same parasite, but at least appear to be concerned with related parasites which, for the time being, can be referred to *Ichthyophonus hoferi*. Inclusion of Sproston's (1944) study here is tentative and suspect, since, as we noted earlier, she attributes several bizarre morphological variations to *I. hoferi* which have not been corroborated by other investigators. Little emphasis will be placed

# Table VI

### Records of *Ichthyophonus* infections of fishes from the North Atlantic[1]

| Species | References |
|---|---|
| *Alosa pseudoharengus* (alewife) | Fish, 1934; Sindermann, 1958 |
| *Aphanopus carbo* (black scabbardfish)[2] | Agius, 1978 |
| *Clupea harengus harengus* (Atlantic herring) | Cox, 1916; Daniel, 1933a; Fish, 1934; Sindermann & Scattergood, 1954; Sindermann, 1956, 1958[3] |
| *Gadus morhua* (Atlantic cod) | Machado-Cruz, 1961; McVicar & McKenzie, 1972; Hendricks, 1972; Möller, 1974 |
| *Limanda ferruginea* (yellowtail flounder) | Powles et al., 1968; Ruggieri et al, 1970; Hendricks, 1972 |
| *Melanogrammus aeglefinus* (haddock) | Robertson, 1909 |
| *Myoxocephalus octodecemspinosus* (longhorn sculpin) | Hendricks, 1972 |
| *Platichthys flesus* (flounder) | Robertson, 1908, 1909 |
| *Pleuronectes platessa* (plaice)[4] | Johnstone, 1906, 1920 |
| *Pollachius virens* (pollock) | Priebe, 1973 |
| *Pseudopleuronectes americanus* (winter flounder) | Ellis, 1928; Fish, 1934 |
| *Salmo trutta* (brown trout; sea trout) | Robertson, 1909 |
| *Scomber scombrus* (Atlantic mackerel) | Johnstone, 1913; Sproston, 1944; Sindermann, 1958 |

[1] To our knowledge, there are no detailed reports from the South Atlantic or any other sea or ocean except the Mediterranean. These records may be found in Reichenbach-Klinke (1956b). Sindermann (1963, 1970) presents information supporting the possibility that *I. hoferi* occurs in the North Pacific.

[2] Reported as an infection cause by an "*Ichthyophonus*-like" fungus.

[3] Sindermann & Scattergood (1954) and Sindermann (1958) have reported successful experimental infections of Atlantic herring, killifish (*Fundulus heteroclitus*), goldfish and the calanoid copepod *Calanus finmarchicus* using material from naturally infected Atlantic herring.

[4] In accordance with Fish (1934), we have doubts concerning the validity of this record for this list although it has been included in other lists of this type (Sindermann & Scattergood, 1954; Johnson & Sparrow, 1961).

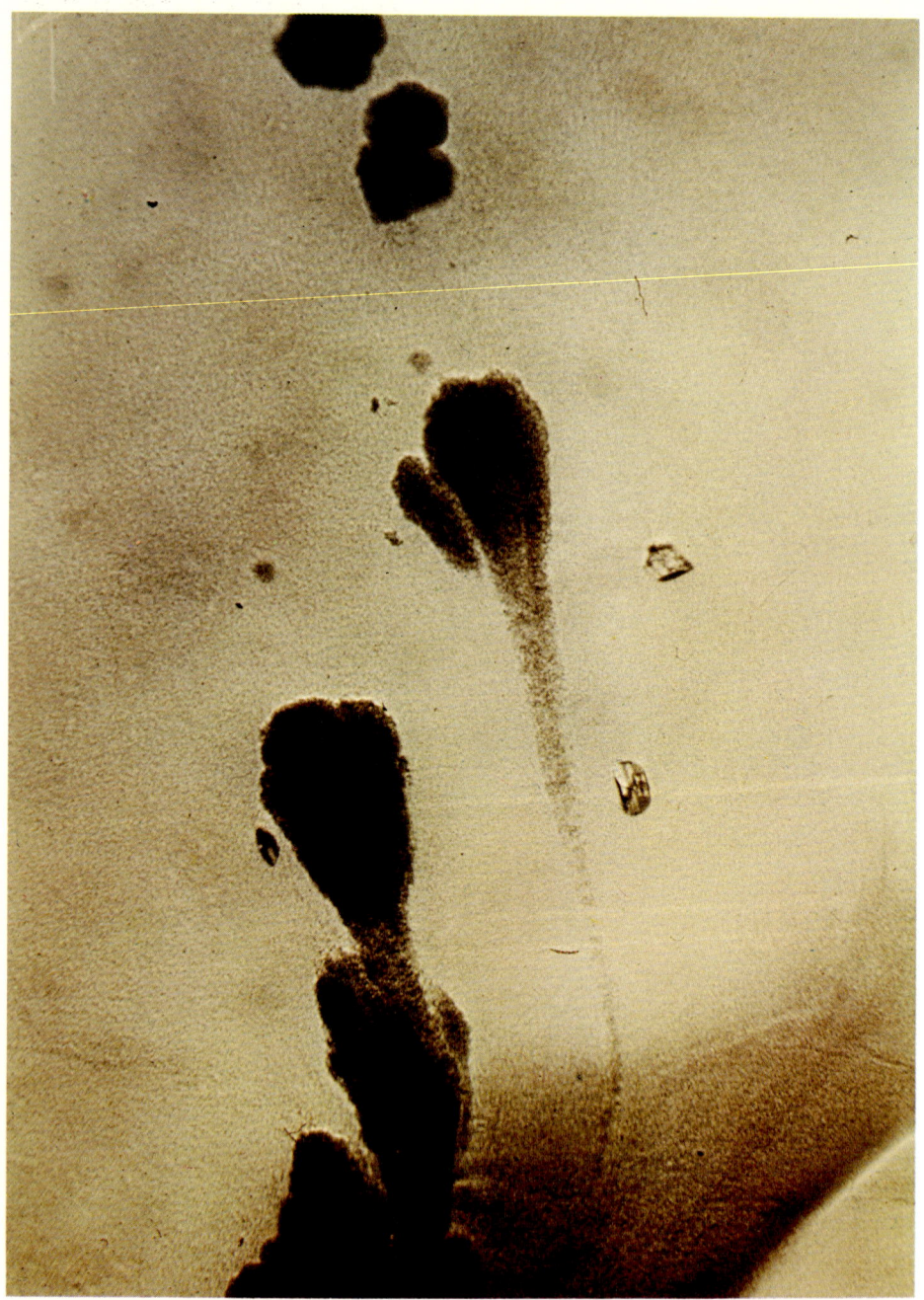

Plate 22. Nutrient agar culture of *Ichthyophonus hoferi* isolated from *Symphysodon axelrodi*. For discussion, see text. (Photograph courtesy of H.-H. Reichenbach-Klinke.)

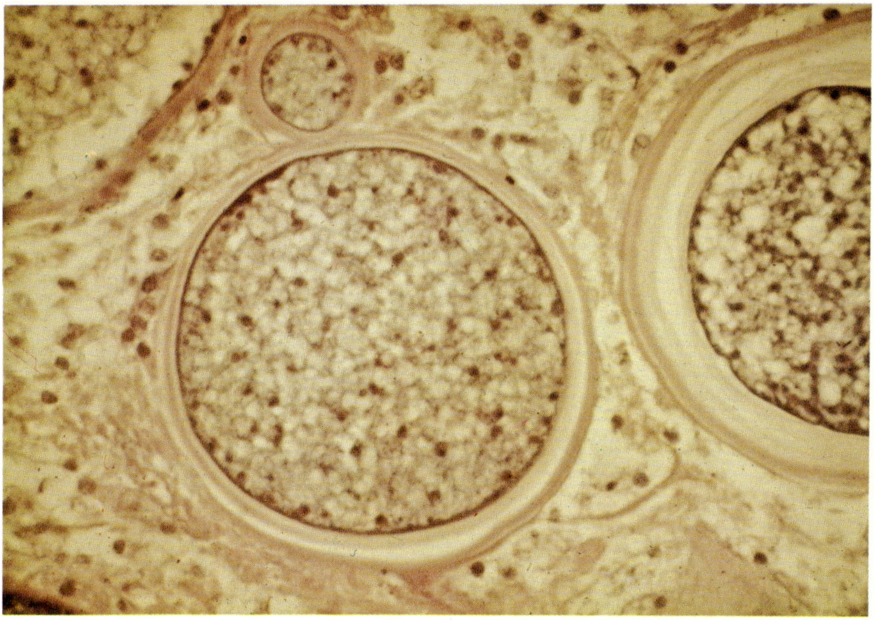

Plate 23. *Ichthyophonus* "resting spores" in the liver of a yellowtail flounder (*Limanda ferruginea*). (Photograph courtesy of Geo. D. Ruggieri and R.F. Nigrelli.)

Plate 24. Chinook salmon (*Oncorhynchus tshawytscha*) fingerling infected by *Phoma herbarum*. Note that the stomach is filled with fluid. (Photograph courtesy of the Western Fish Disease Laboratory, Seattle, Washington.)

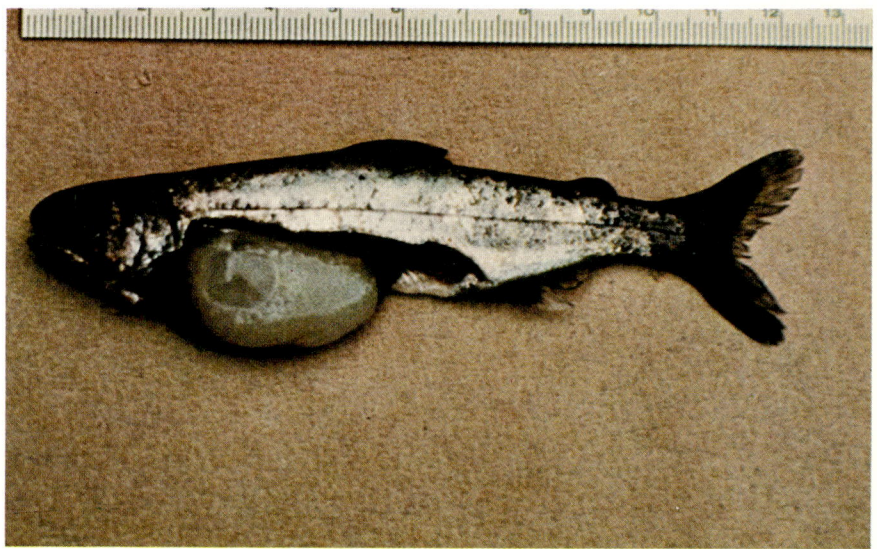

## Table VII
### Records of *Ichthyophonus* infections of freshwater salmonids

| Species | References |
| --- | --- |
| *Oncorhynchus kisutch* (coho salmon) | Gustafson & Rucker, 1956 |
| *Oncorhynchus nerka* (sockeye salmon) | Gustafson & Rucker, 1956 |
| *Oncorhynchus tshawytscha* (chinook salmon) | Gustafson & Rucker, 1956 |
| *Salmo gairdneri* (rainbow trout) | Laveran & Petit, 1910; Plehn & Mulsow, 1911; Pettit, 1913; Neresheimer & Clodi, 1914; Rucker & Gustafson, 1953; Gustafson & Rucker, 1956; Ross & Parisot, 1958; Bellet, 1959; Dorier & Degrange, 1961; Erickson, 1965; Amlacher, 1965 |
| *Salmo trutta* (brown trout) | Neresheimer & Clodi, 1914 |
| *Salvelinus fontinalis* (brook trout) | Pettit, 1913; Neresheimer & Clodi, 1914; Dorier & Degrange, 1961 |

on studies concerned with *Ichthyophonus* infections of freshwater tropical or "aquarium" fishes. This does not mean that we are convinced that these fishes are not susceptible to ichthyophonosis, but we feel that more research is necessary to establish the extent to which true *Ichthyophonus* infections have been confused with granulomatous infections caused by other organisms.

Ichthyophonosis was originally called *Taumelkrankheit* or "reeling disease," in reference to the uncoordinated swimming movements of infected trout as observed by Hofer (1893). However, there are really no external symptoms which can be considered pathognomic for *Ichthyophonus* infections. *I. hoferi* causes systemic granulomatous infections. Whether a fish becomes infected, which organs become infected, the extent of the damage resulting from the proliferation and encystment of the parasite, and the consequent symptoms observed as a reflection of this damage, can vary among different species of fishes and among different individuals of the same species.

Dorier & Degrange (1961) reported that rainbow trout, apparently infected after being fed fresh mackerel, exhibited erratic swimming movements and, occasionally, spiral or "corkscrew" movements consistent with Taumelkrankheit. However, they found that experimentally infected fish died before there was extensive involvement of the central nervous system and therefore did not show these symptoms. Some trout examined by Dorier & Degrange ceased growth and became emaciated whereas others, while heavily infected, could not be distinguished from uninfected fish on the basis of external examination. It is difficult to interpret these findings of Dorier & Degrange. The spiral swimming movements and general loss of equilibrium characteristic of Taumelkrankheit caused by *Ichthyophonus* are also symptomatic of thiamme deficiency disease in fishes. It has been known for some time (see discussions in Snieszko, 1972, and Ashley, 1972) that the flesh of fresh fishes commonly fed to cultured salmonids (brook, brown, and rainbow trout) contains a thiaminase (Krampitz & Woolley, 1944) which hydrolyzes much of the thiamine available in the diets of these animals. Unless fresh food fish are heated to inactivate the enzyme or the diet is supplemented with thiamine, there is a good chance that fishes eating this food will develop thiamine deficiency disease and a characteristic Taumelkrankheit. It is, therefore, most important that nutritional data are also considered in interpreting studies of ichthyophonosis of cultured fishes.

Rucker & Gustafson (1953), who studied ichthyophonosis of rainbow trout from western Washington, found that the fish showed no decrease in appetite or activity during the early stages of the disease and also displayed no peculiar swimming motions. As the disease progressed, the fish became increasingly listless and showed a darkened colour along the lateral line which later became a universal darkening. A swelling of the abdomen as a result of the enlargement of the liver, spleen and kidney was also observed. Rucker & Gustafson reported that infection of the brain was rare. This is in contradistinction to the results reported by Erickson (1965) who found that *Ichthyophonus* infections in the brains of infected rainbow trout from southern Idaho were associated with spinal curvature caused by atrophic musculature pulling the spine out of its normal attitude (see Plates 19, 21). This

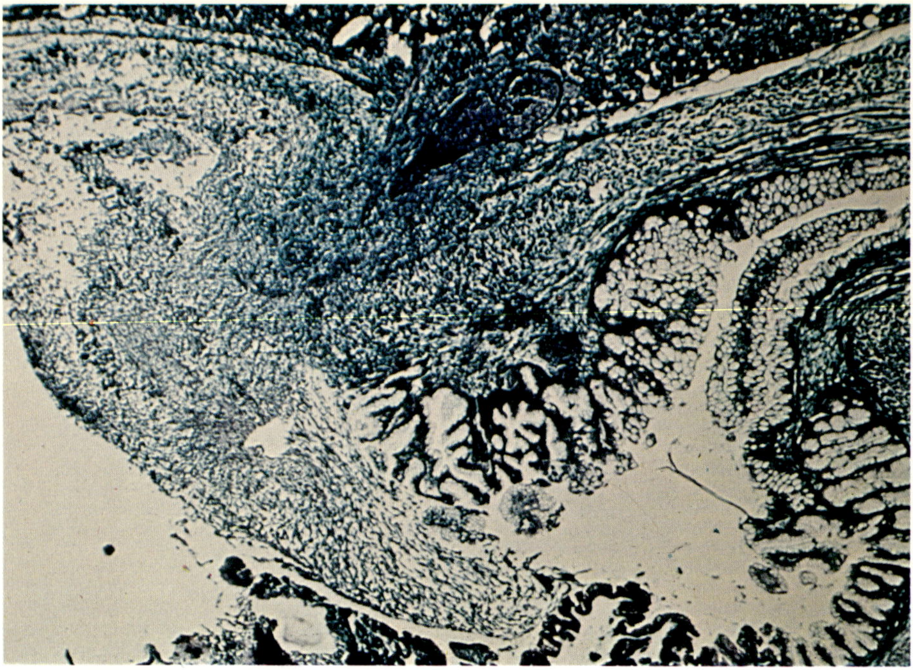

Plate 25. Low magnification photomicrograph of the stomach wall of a fall chinook salmon *(Oncorhynchus tshawytscha)* fingerling experimentally infected by *Phoma herbarum*. Giemsa; X 140. (Photograph courtesy of the Western Fish Disease Laboratory, Seattle, Washington.)

Plate 26. Hyphae of *Phoma herbarum* from the abdominal cavity of a fall chinook salmon *(Oncorhynchus tshawytscha)* fingerling. PAS; x 1300. (Photograph courtesy of the Western Fish Disease Laboratory.)

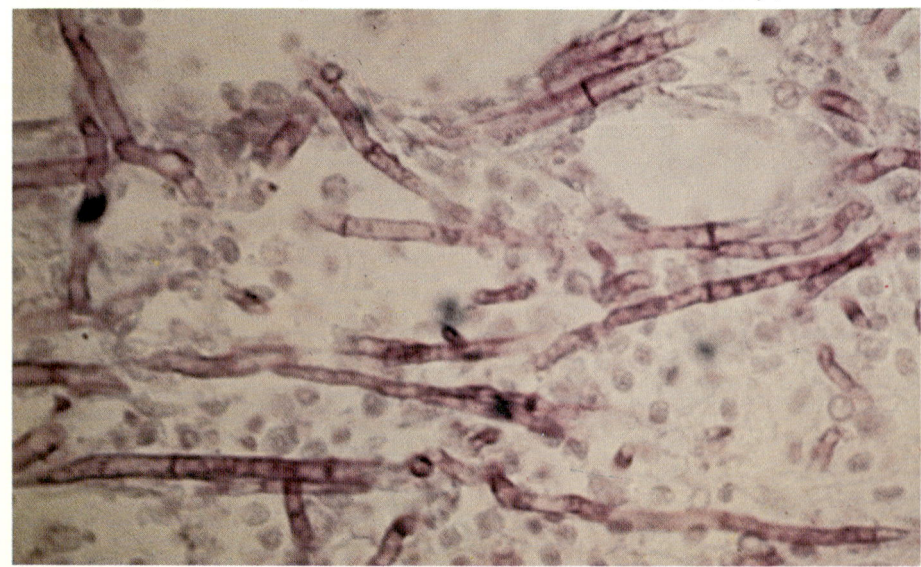

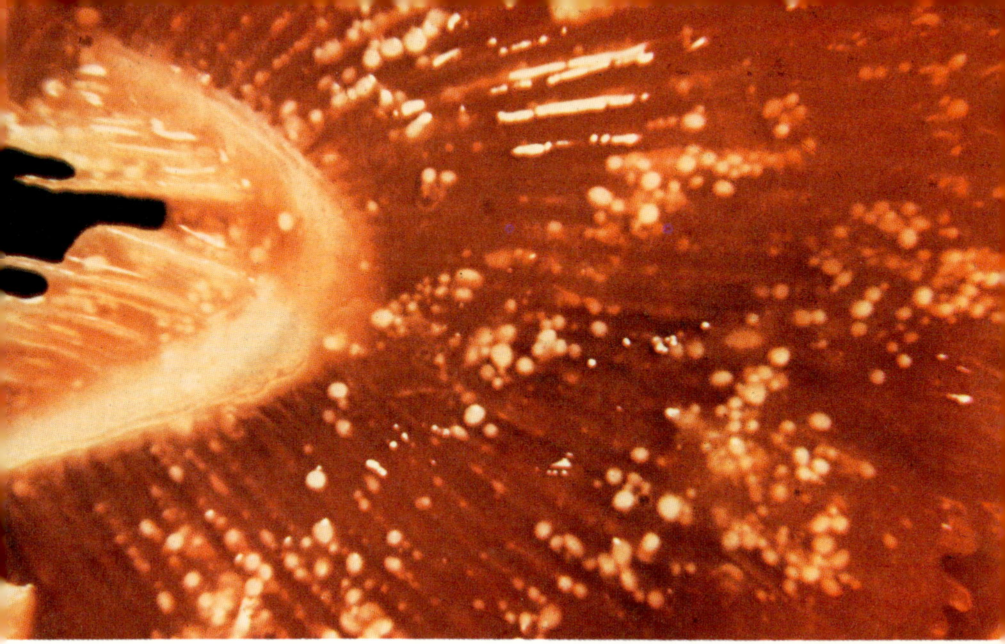

Plate 27. *Dermocystidium* cysts on the gills of a sockeye salmon *(Oncorhynchus nerka)* from the Nimpkish River epizootic (British Columbia). (Photograph courtesy of G.R. Bell and T.P.T. Evelyn.)

Plate 28. Section of the gills of a sockeye salmon (*Oncorhynchus nerka*) showing *Dermocystidium* cysts. PAS-light green. (Photograph courtesy of G.R. Bell and T.P.T. Evelyn.)

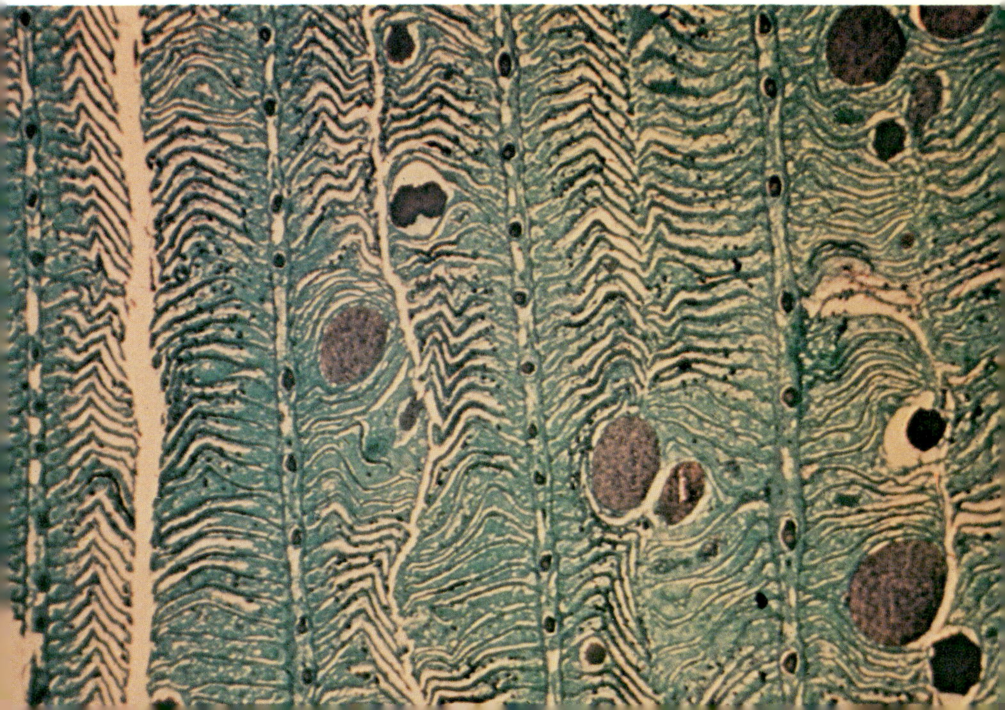

is similar to the sigmoid flexure of the spine noted in some herring (Sindermann & Scattergood, 1954; Sindermann, 1956) which was thought to be the result of infection of the central nervous system, although in rainbow trout such symptoms can also be associated with an ascorbic acid or tryptophan deficiency (Ashley et al., 1975).

Other signs of *Ichthyophonus* infections can be quite varied. In Atlantic herring (Sindermann & Scattergood, 1954), infection of the lateral musculature results eventually in the so-called "sandpaper effect," a roughening of the skin due to the formation of large numbers of papules caused by proliferation of the fungus and the formation of necrotic areas in the subepidermal tissue. Reichenbach-Klinke (1956b) reported blindness and exophthalmos of serranid fish from the Mediterranean as a result of eye infections. This same author (Reichenbach-Klinke, 1960) reported that cranial and dorsal ulcerations *(Lochkrankheit)* are typical of cichlids whereas anabantids display reddening and ulcerations more similar to the Atlantic herring symptoms. Reports of sex reversal (Wurmbach, 1951) and "pathological parthenogenesis" (Stolk, 1958, 1959, 1961) in cyprinodont fishes need to be confirmed.

Dissection of infected fishes will often reveal white, macroscopic, well-defined nodules of connective tissue in the affected organs (Fig. 15). *I. hoferi* elicits a severe focal granulomatous response resulting in cirrhosis and atrophy of the affected organs which can eventually lead to replacement of most of the normal tissue by reticulo-endothelial granulation tissue.

No tissue or organ appears to be immune from infection but, in general, organs with a rich blood supply seem to be more frequently affected, particularly the heart and liver. However, absence of infection of these organs or, for that matter, absence of nodules, does not indicate that the fish is free from infection. In these cases, smears of tissue from likely target organs (e.g. liver, kidney, spleen) may reveal the parasite.

There have been several histopathological studies of *Ichthyophonus* infections. One of the more recent and detailed studies is that of Amlacher (1965) who studied *Ichthyophonus* infections of *Salmo gairdneri*. Amlacher also summarized pertinent aspects of important previous studies including the work by

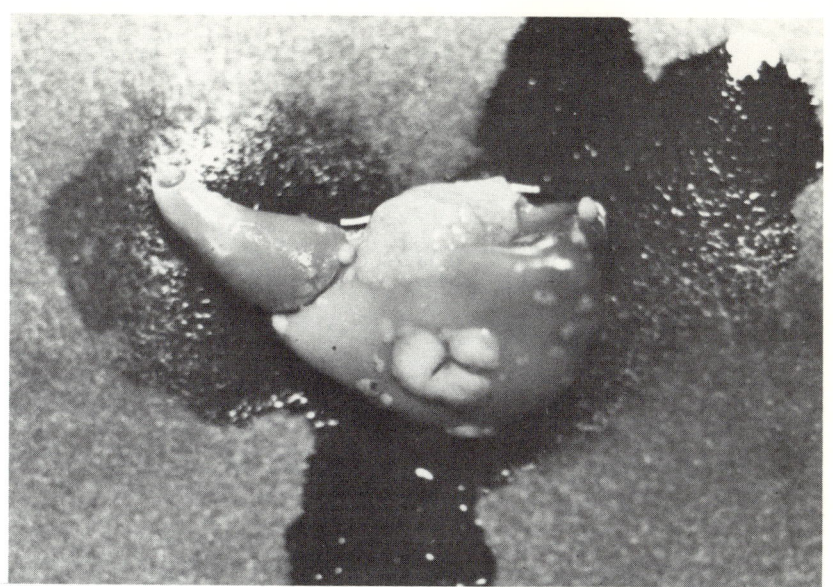

Fig. 15. Nodules on the heart of a yellowtail flounder ( *Limanda ferruginea*) caused by *Ichthyophonus*. (Photograph courtesy of Geo. D. Ruggieri and R.F. Nigrelli.)

Robertson (1908, 1909), Laveran & Pettit (1910), Plehn & Mulsow (1911), Pettit (1913), Neresheimer & Clodi (1914), Daniel (1933a,b), Fish (1934), Sindermann & Scattergood (1954) and Dorier & Degrange (1961).

According to Amlacher, the first tissue response of the host consists of an increased activity of the leucocytes, particularly the eosinophilic granulocytes. These leucocytes surround the parasite and many are destroyed. During this process, fibrocytes appear and eventually enclose (with one to several layers of long cells) the resting spore of the parasite, the leucocytes, and necrotic debris. The result is a characteristic granuloma consisting of the central, thick-walled, multinucleate resting spore surrounded by necrotic cells enclosed within a connective tissue capsule. In other instances the parasite may be surrounded by long, radially arranged cells or by epithelioid cells surrounded by a connective tissue capsule. Giant cells can also be found, particularly in infected kidneys. Empty resting spores often become infiltrated with connective tissue.

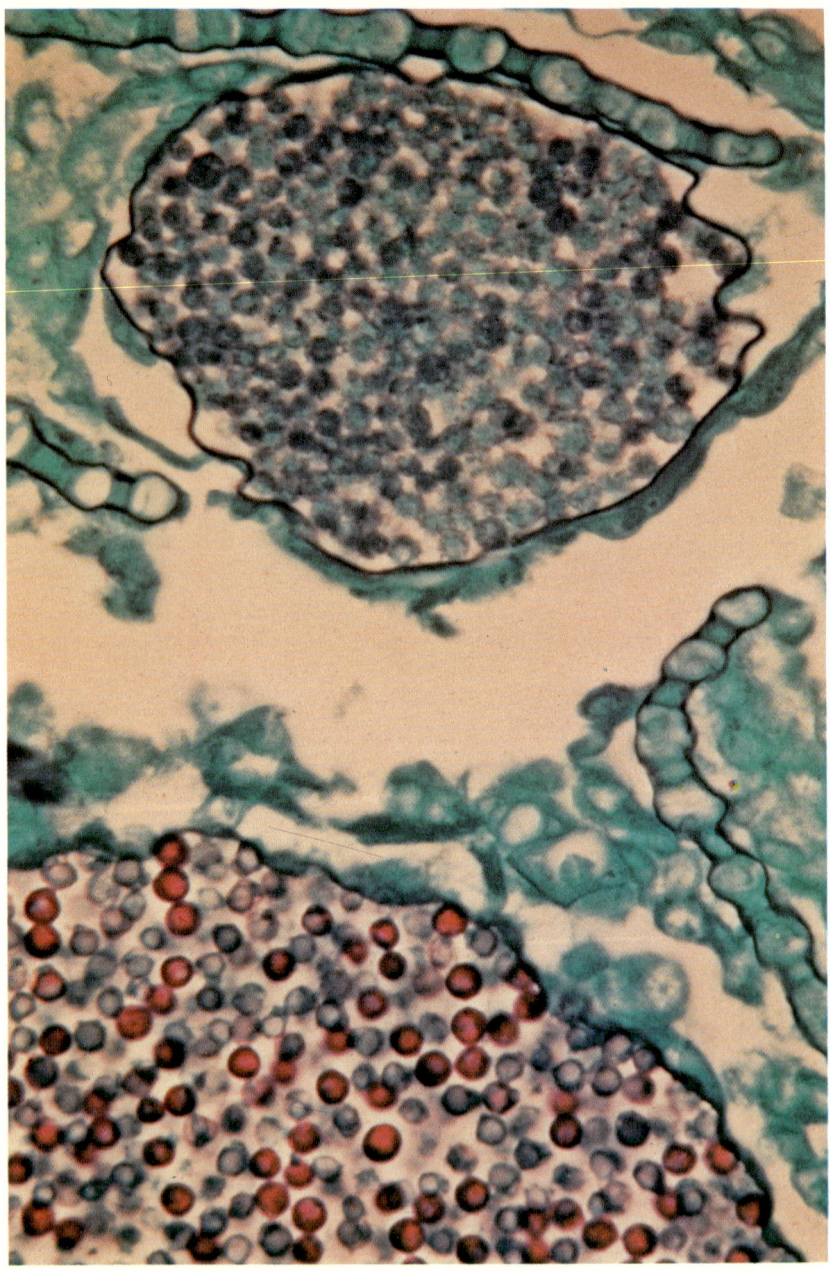

Plate 29. Photomicrograph at a higher magnification of *Dermocystidium* cysts in the gills of a sockeye salmon *(Oncorhynchus nerka)* showing the "spores." PAS-light green. (Photograph courtesy of G.R. Bell and T.P.T Evelyn.)

Several studies have shown that infection is initiated after ingestion of food containing viable *I. hoferi* spores (Pettit, 1913; Neresheimer & Clodi, 1914; Fish, 1934; Gustafson & Rucker, 1956; Sindermann, 1958; Dorier & Degrange, 1961). However, mere ingestion of infectious material does not appear to necessarily ensure infection or, at any rate, serious infection and the factors which promote susceptibility or resistance to infection are poorly understood. An interesting illustration of this is provided by the Atlantic cod (*Gadus morhua*). Recent records (Machado-Cruz, 1961; McVicar & MacKenzie, 1972; Hendricks, 1972; Möller, 1974) have established that the cod is susceptible to *I. hoferi* infections. Möller (1974) found that more than 15% of over 500 fish examined had macroscopically visible nodules and were in significantly poorer condition than uninfected fish. Despite this apparent susceptibility, the epizootic of Atlantic herring in the Gulf of St. Lawrence during 1954-1955, far from having a negative effect on the cod population, was correlated with exceptionally high landings of cod with the increase apparently due to an increase in size of individual fish as a result of the ready availability of dead and dying *I. hoferi*-infected herring as a food source (Sindermann, 1958).

Gustafson & Rucker (1956) found that feeding fresh viscera from infected fish to rainbow trout, three species of Pacific salmon, and a cottid (*Cottus asper*) resulted in infection of these fishes, but they were unable to establish infections in goldfish (*Carassius auratus*), guppies (*Poecilia reticulata*), squawfish (*Ptychocheilus oregonensis*) or brown bullheads (*Ictalurus nebulosus*). Pettit (1913) reported successful experimental infection of tench (*Tinca tinca*), carp (*Cyprinus carpio*) and perch (*Perca fluviatilis*) in addition to numerous successful infections of rainbow trout. Based on their observations of the distribution of the lesions, Gustafson & Rucker (1956) concluded that there could be progressive infection through the wall of the stomach followed by transperitoneal spread through adjacent viscera rather than distribution through the circulatory system. Dorier & Degrange (1961) and Sindermann & Scattergood (1954), on the other hand, believed that the parasite was disseminated by the circulatory system in freshwater salmonids and herring respectively.

Sindermann (1958) also carried out infection experiments with immature Atlantic herring which allowed him to present some quantitative data regarding the dosage required to initiate infection and the relative incidence of acute and chronic infections. He discovered that a single exposure of fifty fish to $2 \times 10^5$ spores resulted in no infection, but several successive exposures to the same dose on successive days did result in infection. Using this information, Sindermann produced an experimental epizootic in 2000 immature Atlantic herring which resulted in infection of 23% of this group—8% acute infections and 15% chronic infections. Mortalities due to acute infections occurred within 2-4 weeks and were characterized by massive invasion of the heart, degeneration and necrosis of the body musculature, and a minimum cellular response from the host. The chronic phase was characterized by a marked host cellular response leading to encapsulation of the parasite by fibrous connective tissue. This was often accompanied by pigment deposition around the "spores" in the muscles. The chronic infections were progressive and terminal in most experimental fish, but a few survived as long as eighteen months.

There are persistent suggestions in the literature that natural *I. hoferi* infections of marine fish may be initiated by ingestion of infected crustaceans, particularly copepods (Jepps, 1937; Reichenbach-Klinke, 1956b; Reichenbach-Klinke & Elkan, 1965; Sindermann & Scattergood, 1954; Sindermann, 1958, 1970); however, definitive evidence of this is lacking.

The most extensive epizootiological studies of *I. hoferi* infections have been concerned with mass mortalities of Atlantic herring in the Gulf of Maine and the Gulf of St. Lawrence. The most recent work on this problem was carried out by C. J. Sindermann who has summarized the results of his investigations in a number of publications (Sindermann, 1956, 1958, 1963, 1966, 1970).

According to Sindermann (1963, 1966), there have been six recorded mass mortalities of herring infected by *I. hoferi*. The first of these is thought to have occurred in 1898 in the Gulf of St. Lawrence and this was followed by another in 1913-1914 (Cox, 1916). On the basis of verbal reports, Sindermann (1963) suggests that the next epizootic occurred in 1940 and this was followed by the most recent one in 1954-1955. The first epizootic in the Gulf of Maine occurred in 1930-1931 (Daniel, 1933a,b; Fish, 1934) and the second occurred in 1947 (Scattergood, 1948), suggesting a 15- to 17-year cycle.

The most extensively documented epizootic is the one which occurred during 1954-1955 and which resulted in the destruction of an estimated one-half of the herring population in the Gulf of St. Lawrence. The first mortalities, which consisted primarily of spring-spawning herring, occurred about mid-May 1954, reached a peak in June, and had apparently ceased by August. This pattern was repeated in 1955, far fewer fish were lost in 1956, and by 1957 no dead herring were found. Subsequent to this epizootic, two strong year-classes in the late 1950's led to an abundant increase in herring stocks up to 1964 but these stocks have declined continuously since then as a result of poor recruitment. Mackerel, on the other hand, as a result of strong year-classes in the mid-1960's, have increased rapidly in abundance and have replaced herring as the dominant pelagic fish in the southern Gulf of St. Lawrence (Winters, 1976).

Powles et al. (1968) and Ruggieri et al. (1970) have presented some epizootiological data for *Ichthyophonus* infections of yellowtail flounder (*Limanda ferruginea*) in the western North Atlantic. Infected fish were first collected in 1966 and again in 1967. Two hundred flounders were collected at each of five collecting sites—the Gulf of St. Lawrence and four sites (Banquereau, Middle Ground, Western Bank, Sable Island Bank) east of Nova Scotia between 43-45°N and 57-62°W. Infected fish were found only in the Western Bank and Sable Island Bank areas which, taken together, gave a mean incidence of infection of about 40%. Fish from the other areas were apparently free from infection. No significant differences in sex ratios or length-weight relationships were found between diseased and normal fish, but fish in the 20-40 cm range appeared to be more susceptible.

The pathological findings for the yellowtail flounders were similar to those previously described (Figs. 11, 15; Plate 23). Fungal lesions were present in the liver, kidney, spleen, body musculature, heart, and gastrointestinal tract. Necrosis was particularly marked in regions associated with germination and hyphal growth. In other areas where resting spores predominated, the fungi became surrounded by reticulo-endothelial cells or by connective tissue fibers. Atrophy with concomitant necrosis was quite evident in the liver, kidney, heart, and body musculature.

Sandholzer, Nostrand & Young (1945) gave epizootiological data for infection of oceanpout, *Macrozoarces americanus*, by an "Ichthyosporidian-like parasite." This work was discussed in some detail by Johnson & Sparrow (1961) as an *I. hoferi* infection, but these authors were apparently not aware of the fact that Nigrelli (1946) had shown that the parasite, now called *Plistophora macrozoarcidis* Nigrelli, is a microsporidian. Similarly, the *Ichthyosporidium* sp. described by Schwartz (1963) as a parasite of *Leiostomus xanthurus* in Chesapeake Bay has been shown by Sprague (1966) to be a microsporidian.

Other epizootics attributed to *I. hoferi* have occurred in trout hatcheries in Europe and North America and, indeed, it should be remembered that *I. hoferi* was first known as a parasite of cultivated salmonids in Europe. However, we know of no reports of epizootics of natural salmonid populations in either Europe or North America. Infection of cultivated fish appears to occur only when these fish have infected raw trash fish included in their diet.

## PREVENTION AND TREATMENT

There is no established chemoprophylactic or chemotherapeutic agent available to deal with *Ichthyophonus* infections. Such agents could not be used in most cases to treat natural populations of marine fishes and it appears that proper hygiene measures, including pasteurization of potentially infected food, will prevent the appearance of the disease in freshwater hatcheries. Since dead and dying fish represent a serious source of contagion, they should be removed and disposed of in accordance with routine hatchery practice. This procedure has also been recommended for natural epizootics, but, in the long run, this may prove to be an unwarranted tampering with nature and could prove to be economically counterproductive as well, since the decimation of one species may allow another, more desirable, species to flourish.

# FUNGI IMPERFECTI

Species of imperfect fungi (Deuteromycetes) are not typically thought of as potential parasites of fish; however, in recent years it has become increasingly clear that such infections, while rare and usually of sporadic occurrence and low incidence, are more common than previously suspected (Table VIII). In fact, some species (*Exophiala salmonis, Exophiala pisciphila, Ochroconis tshawytschae*), as their specific epithets indicate, were first described as fish pathogens. However, it must be noted that these fungi cannot, in any sense, be regarded as specific, or obligate pathogens. Like the saprolegnian fungi, these fungi are facultative necrotrophs in the sense of Cooke (1977). It seems probable that records of infections caused by imperfect fungi will continue to increase in proportion to the incidence of alert and well-trained fish pathologists. We are fortunate, however, that these infections are not more common because they are usually fatal for the affected fish and, at present, there is no practical way to predict, prevent, or treat them.

## Blastomycetes

This group includes ascomycetous and basidiomycetous yeasts for which sexual reproduction has not been demonstrated. *Candidia albicans*, a well known opportunistic pathogen of man, is included in this group and, until just recently, *Cryptococcus neoformans*, another human pathogen, was also included in this group. *C. neoformans* is now known to be a basidiomycete and its "perfect" or sexual stage is called *Filobasidiella neoformans* (Kwon-Chung, 1976)[1]. Further information on the Blastomycetes and pertinent references may be found in the review by Kreger-van Rij (1973).

---

[1]The Fungi Imperfecti are the only group of organisms in which a species can, at the same time, have two or more valid scientific names—one for the "perfect" (sexual) state and one or more for the imperfect (asexual) states. In recent literature the neologisms "teleomorph" and "anamorph" are replacing the terms "perfect state" and "imperfect state" respectively.

## Table VIII

### Fungi Imperfecti reported as fish parasites.

| Fungi | Hosts | References |
|---|---|---|
| **BLASTOMYCETES** | | |
| *Candida sake* (Saito & Ota) van Uden & Buckley | *Oncorhynchus rhodurus* | Hatai & Egusa, 1975 |
| *Cryptococcus* sp. | *Tinca tinca* | Pierotti, 1971 |
| **HYPHOMYCETES** | | |
| *Aureobasidium* sp.[1] | *Trygon pastinacea* | Otte, 1964 |
| | *Cyprinus carpio* | |
| ? *Exophiala* sp.[2] | *Amphiprion sebae* | Blazer & Wolke, 1978 |
| | *Fundulus heteroclitus* | |
| | *Gadus morhua* | |
| | *Hippocampus erectus* | |
| | *Pseudopleuronectes americanus* | |
| | *Stenotomus chrysops* | |
| | *Tautogolabrus adspersus* | |
| | *Xanthichthys ringens* | |

[1] A tentative identification cited as a fungus related to the genus *Pullularia*. *Pullularia* is a synonym of *Aureobasidium*.

[2] Defined by Ajello (1975) as fungi which cause "phaeohyphomycoses" which refers to Fungi Imperfecti or Ascomycetes which "... develop in the host's tissues in the form of dark-walled, septate, mycelial elements."

| Fungi | Hosts | References |
|---|---|---|
| *Exophiala salmonis* Carmichael[2] | *Salmo clarki* Salmo salar Salvelinus namaycush Ictalurus punctatus | Carmichael, 1966; Richards, Holliman & Helgason, 1978; Holliman & Richards, 1978 Fijan, 1969; McGinnis & Ajello, 1974a |
| *Exophiala pisciphila* McGinnis & Ajello[2] | *Cyprinus carpio* | Hörter, 1960 |
| *Fusarium culmorum* (W.G. Smith) Saccardo[3] | | |
| *Ochroconis humicola* (Barron & Busch) de Hoog & von Arx[2] | *Oncorhynchus kisutch* Salmo gairdneri | Ross & Yasutake, 1973; de Hoog & Von Arx, 1973; Ajello, 1975; Ajello, McGinnis & Camper, 1977 |
| *Ochroconis tshawytscha* (Doty & Slater) Kirilenko & All-Achmed[2] | *Oncorhynchus tshawytscha* | Doty & Slater, 1946; McGinnis & Ajello, 1974b, 1975; Kirilenko & All-Achmed, 1977 |
| *Verticillium piscis* (Batista & Maia) Charmichael[4] | *Carassius auratus* | Batista & Maia, 1959 |
| **COELOMYCETES** | | |
| *Phoma herbarum* Westendorp[2] | *Oncorhynchus kisutch* Oncorhynchus tshawytscha Salmo gairdneri | Ross, Yasutake & Leek, 1975; Wolke, 1975; Wood, 1974 |

[3] Cited as *Fusarium culmorum* (W.G. Sm.) Sacc. var. *cereale* (Cke.) Wr., a variety not recognized as distinct from *F. culmorum* by Booth (1971).

[4] Originally named *Gibellulopsis piscis* Batista & Maia. According to Carmichael in Kendrick & Carmichael (1973), *Gibellulopsis* is a synonym of *Verticillium*.

It is not unusual for yeasts, including potential pathogens like *Candida albicans*, to occur as commensals on the surfaces of clinically healthy animals, and fish are no exception. For example, Bruce & Morris (1973) obtained isolates of the genera *Candida, Cryptococcus, Rhodotorula, Torulopsis, Trichosporon,* and *Debaryomyces* from marine fish near Scotland. All these genera, except *Debaryomyces* (an ascomycetous yeast), are classified as Blastomycetes. However, yeast infections of fish are virtually unknown. Pierotti (1971) found a *Cryptococcus* species in association with bilateral exophthalmos of tench and Hatai & Egusa (1975) reported *Candida sake* in association with tympanites of amago salmon (*Oncorhynchus rhodurus*). Wood, Yasutake & Lehman (1955) reported that a yeast was associated with a visceral granuloma of trout, but subsequent work (Landolt, 1975) has failed to confirm a fungal etiology. There appears to be a correlation between diet and the incidence of these granulomas, but the exact etiology is not fully understood. Pauley (1967) reported that he had found a "fungal or yeast-like form" in the testes of salmon but this report needs to be confirmed. Roberts et al. (1973) reported that they had found yeast cells associated with a tagging wound in a salmon, but there appears to be no evidence that these yeasts were, in any sense, pathogens.

## Hyphomycetes

The Hyphomycetes are a diverse assemblage of fungi characterized as mycelial forms which are either sterile or bear conidia (asexual spores) on hyphae or aggregations of hyphae which are not contained within a discrete fructification. Most fungi in this group, including the ones discussed in this volume, are thought to be imperfect forms of Ascomycetes whose perfect state has either not been discovered or no longer exists. Fungi in this group are classified according to morphology, color and arrangement of spores and hyphae, and by the way in which the conidia are produced by the conidiogenous cells. Further information, and a more rigorous definition of these fungi, may be found in Kendrick & Carmichael (1973). An important point to remember is that these fungi are arranged in artificial groups. This point is sometimes emphasized by the use of the terms "form-genus" and "form-species" when referring to them. This means that we cannot automatically assume that there is necessarily a closer phyletic relationship between two form-species in the same form-genus than there is between two form-species placed in different form genera.

On several occasions Hyphomycetes have been found in fish tumours and granulomas, but often it is uncertain whether these are caused by the fungus or whether the fungus is taking advantage of the situation. This aspect of hyphomycete infections has been discussed by Reichenbach-Klinke (1955, 1956d, 1973) who also refers to the significant earlier literature (Montpellier & Dieuzeide, 1932; Harant & Vernierès, 1933; Walker, 1951; Ermin, 1952). Recently Miyazaki & Egusa (1972, 1973a,b,c) have published a series of papers on "mycotic granulomatosis." These papers are written entirely in Japanese and we have not yet been able to evaluate them. Another recently described "mycotic granulomatosis" (Hatai et al., 1977) appears to be caused by an as yet unidentified oomycete.

Often Hyphomycetes are recognized in tumours or granulomas by the presence of septate hyphae and spores, but are not identified further. In the following discussion we will concentrate on those hyphomycete infections from which the fungus has been identified (Table VIII).

## *AUREOBASIDIUM*

Otte (1964) has described an infection of a stingray (*Trygon pastinacea* = *Dasyatis pastinaca*) caused by a fungus which can probably be included in the genus *Aureobasidium* (= *Pullularia*). The infected fish was obtained from a marine aquarium.

The fungus infection was apparently confined to the liver and, apart from some enlargement of the spleen and the presence of a few encysted nematode larvae in the intestine, no other pathological conditions were noted in the other organs.

Gross signs of infection included ascites, swelling of the liver, and the presence of scattered, poorly defined foci whose center consisted of a soft greyish-white mass. Microscopic examination showed that these necrotic foci consisted of cellular debris, fat deposits, and septate hyphae. Histological examination indicated both an acute nonproliferative and a chronic granulomatous response. Pure cultures of the fungus were easily obtained by streaking material from the lesions onto Sabouraud's agar, blood agar, or glucose blood agar.

Successful infection experiments were carried out by intraperitoneal injection of a fungal suspension into two carp weighing 1.5 kg each. The fish were maintained in water with a temperature of 16-20°C and both fish died about a month after injection. The lesions in the carp were similar to those observed in the stingray and the fungus could be re-isolated in pure culture, thus fulfilling Koch's postulates. Unfortunately, there is no record of any isolate being placed in a culture collection so that it would be available to other investigators for further taxonomic or pathological investigations.

## *EXOPHIALA*

Despite the fact that the genus *Exophiala* has been the subject of recent taxonomic scrutiny (McGinnis, 1977; McGinnis & Padhye, 1977; de Hoog, 1977), it remains a taxonomically difficult genus whose representatives cannot be distinguished by the nonspecialist. Formerly defined as a genus that produces a conidiogenous cell called a phialide, it has recently been redefined as a genus which produces its conidia predominantly on another type of conidiogenous cell called an annellide. Of the species presently recognized in this genus, two have been isolated as parasites of fishes — *E. salmonis* Carmichael and *E. pisciphila* McGinnis & Ajello (Fig. 16). Some morphological and physiological features of the isolates of these two species obtained from fishes are given in Table IX. The *Exophiala*-like hyphomycete recently described by Blazer & Wolke (1978) is similar to *E. jeanselmei* (Langeron) McGinnis & Padhye (R.D. Goos and G.A. Neish, unpublished observations) but further work must be carried out on this isolate before any definitive assignment can be made. De Hoog (1977) recognizes several varieties of *E. jeanselmei*.

Carmichael (1966) described three epizootics attributed to *E. salmonis* from a single hatchery in Calgary, Alberta. The first two, which occurred in the winter of 1948-1949 and in December, 1956, respectively, affected young cutthroat trout (*Salmo clarki*). The third occurred in November, 1960 and affected yearling lake trout (*Salvelinus namaycush*). The gross symptoms of the infections were not pathognomic. The fish exhibited ataxia and erratic

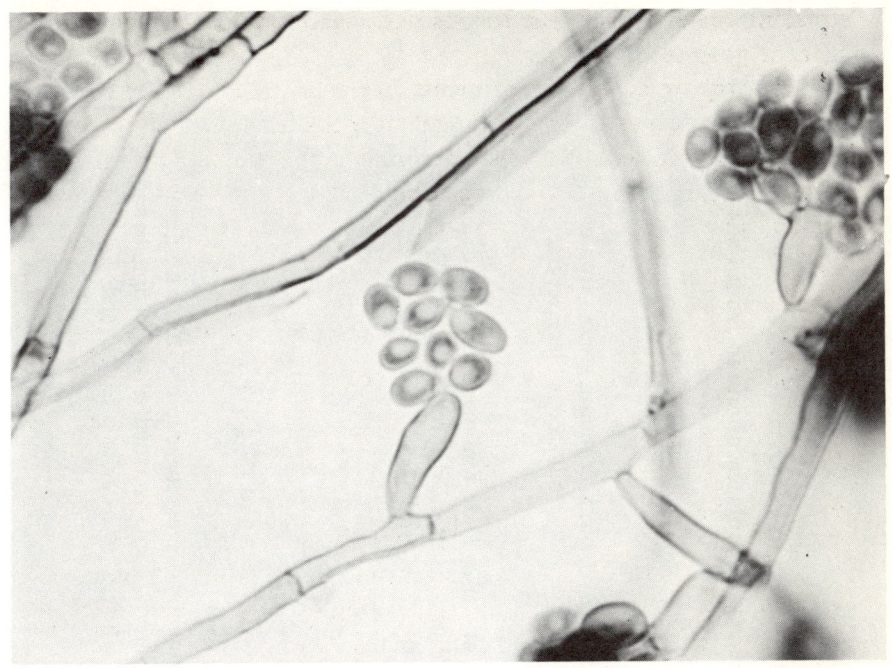

Fig. 16. *Exophiala pisciphila* McGinnis & Ajello showing conidiogenous cells and conidia. X 1900. (Photograph courtesy of L. Ajello.)

swimming movements, followed by whirling movements, exophthalmos, and the formation of cranial ulcers followed by death. In the first epizootic the incidence of infection may have been as high as 40%; estimates were not given for the other epizootics. Attempts to obtain experimental infections by exposure to heavy spore suspensions or by intraperitoneal, intramuscular, intracranial or subcutaneous injection were unsuccessful.

Histological examination showed a chronic granulomatous response with the presence of many giant cells. Necrotic areas with extensive hyphal development could also be observed. The lesions were confined to the brain; *E. salmonis* could not be demonstrated in the eyes, gills, lower jaw or any internal organs.

Carmichael (1966) referred to the infection of the salmonids by *E. salmonis* as a "cerebral mycetoma"; however, both Ajello (1975) and Wolke (1975) have apparently independently concluded that the use of the term "mycetoma" is inaccurate since the fungus was not organized in the form of granules. Ajello (1975)

# TABLE IX

## Comparison of some morphological and physiological features of the *Exophiala salmonis* and *Exophiala pisciphila* isolates obtained from fishes.[1]

| | *E. salmonis* | *E. pisciphila* |
|---|---|---|
| **COLONY** | | |
| colour | mouse grey with darker grey reverse | blackish mouse grey to iron grey with olivaceous black reverse. |
| growth 25°C | 5-8 mm diameter in 14 da on cellophane on Czapek's, cereal or PYE agar | 25-28 mm diameter in 14 da on potato-dextrose, cereal or V-8 juice juice agar |
| 37°C | no growth | no growth |
| **ANNELLOCONIDIA** | | |
| colour | yellow-brown | yellow-brown |
| shape | cylindrical clavate with distal end rounded; proximal end slightly stipitate with a flat scar; constricted at septum | subglobose to obovoid with distal end rounded; slightly stipitate and truncate at proximal end |

| | | |
|---|---|---|
| septation | 0-2 septate; typically 1-septate with a heavy refractile septum | aseptate |
| size | septate conidia 3 X 11-14 microns; aseptate conidia 3 X 5-8 microns | 2-3 X 3-5 microns |
| SPORULATION | good on cereal or cornmeal agar; poor or absent on PYE or Sabouraud's agar | good on potato-dextrose, cereal and V-8 agar; poor on Sabouraud's agar |

[1] Based on data given in Carmichael (1966) and McGinnis & Ajello (1974a). For more expanded descriptions of these species, see de Hoog (1977).

also found *E. salmonis* infections in a hatchery in North Carolina but no details were given.

The most recent records of *E. salmonis* infections of fishes are those by Richards, Holliman & Helgason (1978) and Holliman & Richards (1978) who studied naturally occurring and experimentally induced infections of Atlantic salmon (*Salmo salar*). The results of these studies were not available to us as this volume goes to press so we have not been able to evaluate them.

The sole epizootic attributed to *Exophiala pisciphila* occurred among channel catfish (*Ictalurus punctatus*) in a small pond in Alabama (Fijan, 1969). Gross symptoms included round or irregular external ulcers 2-15 mm in diameter, soft nodules of varying size in the viscera, absence of a serous membrane on the surface of the nodules, and the presence of an exudate. Histological examination confirmed the presence of both an acute non-proliferative response and a chronic proliferative granulomatous response.

Fungal hyphae were easily isolated from the nodules and attempts to reproduce the infections by intraperitoneal injection with a fungal suspension were successfully carried out using three species of fishes (*Ictalurus punctatus, Ictalurus catus, Lepomis macrochirus*). The first experimentally infected fish died within 13 days and all fish were dead within a month.

Blazer & Wolke (1978) have discussed naturally occurring infections of several species of fishes from an aquarium in Mystic, Connecticut caused by an *Exophiala*-like fungus (Table VIII). These authors also obtained successful experimental infections of three species of fishes (*Fundulus heteroclitus, Pseudopleuronectes americanus, Tautogolabrus adspersus*) by intraperitoneal injections with spore suspensions.

Two naturally infected fishes (*Hippocampus erectus, Xanthichthys ringens*) examined by Blazer & Wolke had non-ulcerated external dermal masses present as a result of the fungal infection and gross internal lesions were found in two naturally infected fishes (*Gadus morhua, Stenotomus chrysops)* and one experimentally infected fish (*T. adspersus*). In the natural cases, these internal lesions consisted of raised, round, yellow to white areas on several organs. In the *T. adspersus*, yellowish depressed to level lesions were found on the liver only.

Blazer & Wolke found that the inflammatory reaction could be either an acute nonproliferative or a chronic proliferative response. These authors divided the acute response into two types. The first, which consisted of necrosis with the presence of pale eosinophilic granulocytes and macrophages, was the more common in the naturally occurring infections. The second type, which consisted of necrosis with little inflammatory response, was found in fishes experimentally injected with a spore suspension. In both cases, hyphae could usually be distinguished in the tissues. The most interesting chronic inflammatory response was found in a naturally infected *Gadus morhua*. This reaction was characterized by focal granulomas which were multiple with a central zone of caseous necrosis of calcification surrounded by epithelioid cells. This reaction closely resembled piscine mycobacteriosis and, once again, demonstrated the difficulties that can be encountered in differential diagnosis.

## *FUSARIUM CULMORUM*

Hörter (1960) reported a curious case where two hundred carp transplanted to a newly constructed earthen pond died within a few weeks from fungal invasion of the eyes and skin. The causative agent was identified as *Fusarium culmorum* var. *cereale* (See *footnote 3*, Table VIII). Hörter was of the opinion that a heavy covering of beech (*Fagus* sp.) leaves on the bottom of the pond provided the substrate for massive development of the fungus which was able to act as an opportunistic parasite of carp subjected to severe environmental stress.

## *OCHROCONIS*

Two species belonging to the genus *Ochroconis (O. humicola* and *O. tshawytschae)* have been found as parasites of fishes. These two species were formerly placed in the better known genus *Scolecobasidium* Abbott 1927 but recent taxonomic studies by de Hoog & von Arx (1973) and by Kirilenko & All-Achmed (1977) have resulted in the transfer of these species to the newly created genus *Ochroconis* de Hoog & von Arx 1973. *Ochroconis* species produce an ellipsoidal to cylindrical sympodioconidium with a broadly rounded tip and a conspicuous hilum at the base which marks the point of attachment to a denticle on the conidiogenous cell (Fig. 17).

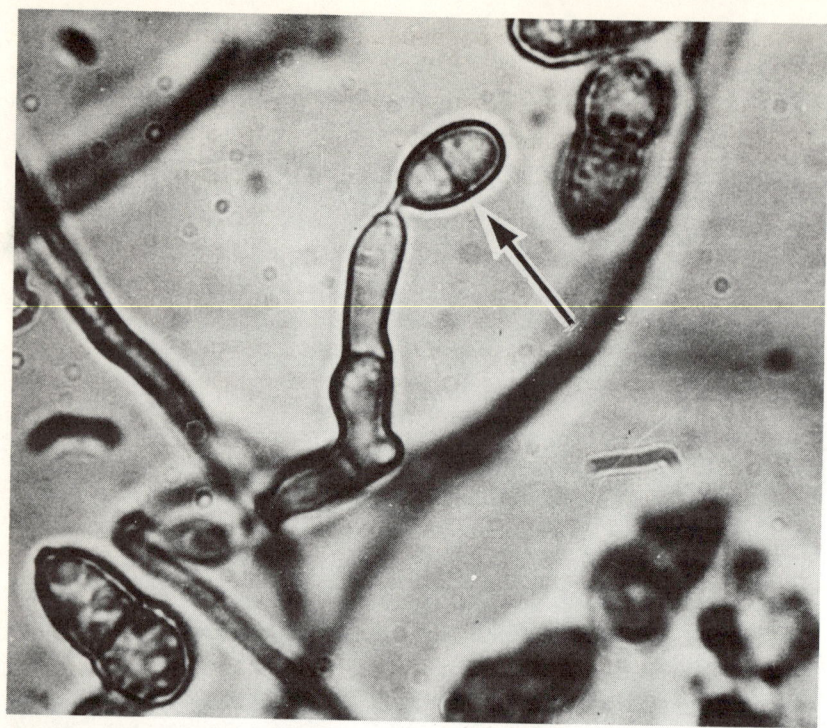

Fig. 17. Slide culture of *Ochroconis humicola*, showing immature septate conidium (arrow). X 3140. (Photograph courtesy of A. J. Ross and W. T. Yasutake, with permission of the Journal of the Fisheries Research Board of Canada.)

## *Ochroconis humicola*

This organism was originally described from soil (Barron & Busch, 1962) and has subsequently been regarded as a possible pathogen of frogs (Elkan & Philpot, 1973) and as a pathogen of young coho salmon (Ross & Yasutake, 1973) and rainbow trout (Ajello, 1975; Ajello, McGinnis & Camper, 1977). On potato dextrose agar the colonies reach a diameter of about 40 mm at 25°C and are olive coloured with a dark brown to olivaceous black reverse. No growth occurs at 37°C. The conidiophores occasionally become comparatively long (up to 300 microns), septate, undulating and intertwining, but are usually much shorter (5-30 microns). The conidia are usually one-septate, ovoid to short cylindric, finely echinulate, average 3.5 X 10 microns, and taper to a narrow connective corresponding to the attachment point (Fig. 17).

*O. humicola* caused only a low incidence of infection in the salmon (Ross & Yasutake, 1973) and attempts to establish experimental infections were successful only when fungal inoculum was fed to the fish with a dry meal diet containing ground glass. Even then, infection could be demonstrated in only three of ten experimental fish.

Foci of infection were particularly evident in the kidney, but *O. humicola* could also infect other organs and could cause external lesions (Fig. 18). Internal gross lesions included ascites, frequent adhesions, and grey areas in the organs which could be confused with those seen in cases of corynebacterial kidney infections. Histological examination showed numerous large lesions infiltrated with hyphae and lymphoid cells (Fig. 19). Foci of degeneration and necrosis were often observed as well, but no giant cells were found.

Ajello, McGinnis & Camper (1977) have recently described *O. humicola* infections of rainbow trout at a hatchery in Tennessee. Outbreaks occurred each autumn from 1969 to 1973 and then ceased when the hatchery water supply (which was contaminated with seepage from a septic tank) was changed.

Fig. 18. External lesion on a coho salmon (*Oncorhynchus kisutch*) caused by *Ochroconis humicola*. (Photograph courtesy of A. J. Ross and W. T. Yasutake, with permission of the Journal of the Fisheries Research Board of Canada.)

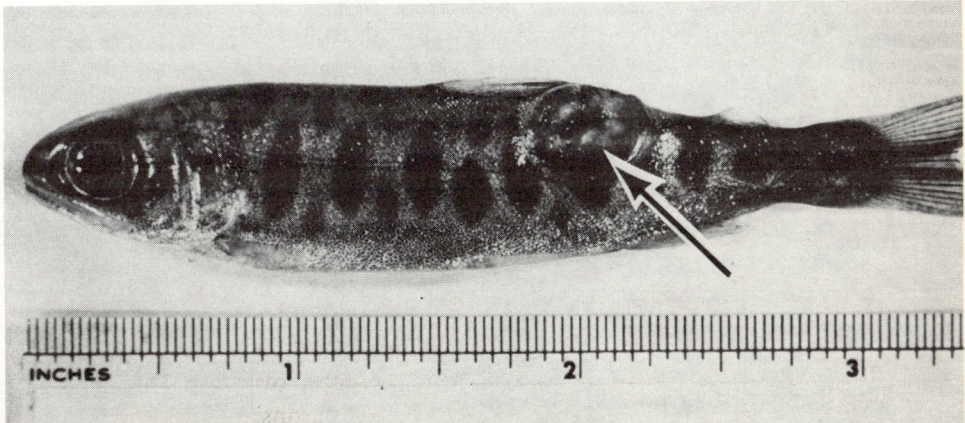

The infected fish exhibited a variety of gross external and internal lesions. External lesions included blister-like areas, ulcerations, and hemorrhage and anemia of the gills. Edema and exophthalmos were also noted. Internally there was hemorrhage throughout the body cavity and the frequent occurrence of clumps of dematiaceous mycelium. The kidneys were swollen and bathed in a bloody fluid and the liver and spleen were hemorrhagic and pale. Histologic examination showed abundant hyphae and a granulomatous reaction characterized by infiltration of lymphocytes and mononuclear cells. Progressive replacement of normal tissue by granulation was observed in the kidneys.

Yearling rainbow trout were easily infected experimentally by intraperitoneal injections with a suspension of *O. humicola* hyphae and spores. Tissue invasion occurred within three days and the fish generally died 7 to 10 days after the injections.

Fig. 19. Histopathological changes occurring in the peripheral area of the external lesion on coho salmon caused by *Ochroconis humicola* and shown in Figure 18. Note hyphae and widespread inflammation in the infected area. May-Gruenwald stain, X 825. (Photograph courtesy of A. J. Ross and W. T. Yasutake, with permission of the Journal of the Fisheries Research Board of Canada.)

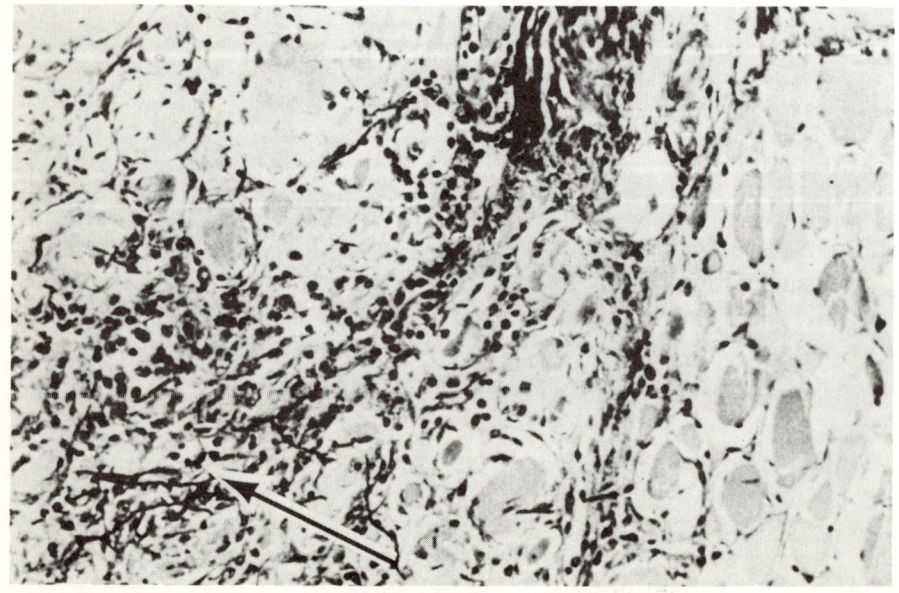

## *Ochroconis tshawytschae*

This species has a somewhat complex taxonomic history so its complete synonymy is given in the following list:
= *Ochroconis tshawytschae* (Doty & Slater) Kirilenko & All-Achmed 1977. Mikrobiol. Zh. 39: 303-306.
= *Heterosporium tshawytschae* Doty & Slater, 1946. Am. Midl. Nat. 36: 663.
= *Scolecobasidium macrosporum* Roy, Dwivedi & Mishra, 1962. Lloydia 25: 164-166.
= *Scolecobasidium variabile* Barron & Busch, 1962. Can. J. Bot. 40: 83-84.
= *Scolecobasidium tshawytschae* (Doty & Slater) McGinnis & Ajello, 1974. Trans. Br. mycol. Soc. 63: 202-203.

*O. tshawytschae* has been isolated from soil (Barron & Busch, 1962; Roy, Dwivedi & Mishra, 1962) and from the surface of tomato roots (Kirilenko & All-Achmed, 1977), but was originally isolated as a pathogen of young chinook salmon (Doty & Slater, 1946). On potato dextrose agar the colonies reach a diameter of 20-40 mm in three weeks at 25°C and are olive coloured with a dark olive reverse. *O. tshawytschae* can be distinguished from other species in the genus by its capacity to produce three-septate, ovoid to cylindric, minutely echinulate conidia. The average size of the conidium is about 3.5 X 14 microns.

*O. tshawytschae* was isolated from the kidneys of chinook salmon yearlings at the Colemen Fisheries Station, Anderson, California, in 1946. According to Doty & Slater (1946) the infections were usually found in the posterior half of the kidneys and were usually localized in two or three foci. These authors believed that the first part of the kidneys to become infected were the mesonephric tubules and they suggested that the mesonephric ducts from the cloaca provided the route of entry for the pathogen. Less than one percent of the fish were infected and the disease did not appear to be very infectious.

This is apparently the only incidence of infection of an animal attributed to *O. tshawytschae* and no further efforts have been made to establish its potential pathogenicity.

## VERTICILLIUM PISCIS

Originally described as *Gibellulopsis piscis* in 1959, this organism was thought to be the cause of a granuloma in a goldfish. Carmichael (Kendrick & Carmichael, 1973) has noted that *Gibellulopsis* Batista & Maia is a synonym of *Verticillium* Nees, but otherwise this organism has been generally ignored by both mycologists and fish pathologists.

## Coelomycetes

The Coelomycetes differ from the Hyphomycetes by the fact that their conidia are produced in some type of fructification, the three basic types being pycnidia (Fig. 20), acervuli and stromata. *Phoma herbarum* Westend., the type species of a genus comprised of hundreds of species, is the only coelomycete reported as a fish parasite. It produces hyaline, usually 4.5-5.0 X 2.0-2.5 microns aseptate, elliptical to oval conidia in simple or compound pycnidia (Fig. 20). These fructifications are not produced *in vivo* but are usually readily produced *in vitro*.

*P. herbarum* must be grown in culture to establish its identity. It grows well on a wide variety of standard mycological media such as cornmeal agar, oatmeal agar, potato dextrose agar, and malt agar. Ross, Yasutake & Leek (1975) reported that they could usually obtain pure cultures by inoculating material from the abdominal cavity of infected fish directly onto Sabouraud's dextrose agar. Further information on *P. herbarum* in particular may be found in Boerema (1964, 1970) and on Coelomycetes in general in Sutton (1973).

*Phoma herbarum* infections have been found in three species of salmonids (*Oncorhynchus kisutch, Oncorhynchus tshawytscha, Salmo gairdneri*) in the northwestern United States. According to Ross, Yasutake & Leek (1975) spring chinook salmon appear to be the most severely affected with losses as high as 2.6% having been reported from the Little White Salmon hatchery in Washington. The disease is usually found in fish less than 100 days old and the infections appear to be initiated in the air bladder. This has led Wood (1974) to postulate that infection might occur during the "swim up" stage at the time of the initial filling of the air bladder.

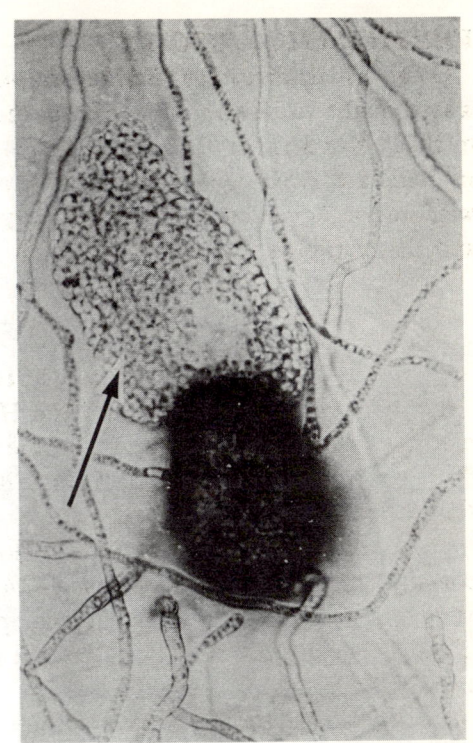

Fig. 20. Slide culture of *Phoma herbarum* showing conidia extruded from ruptured pycnidium. X 625. (Photograph courtesy of A. J. Ross, W. T. Yasutake, and S. Leek, with permission of the Journal of the Fisheries Research Board of Canada.)

This hypothesis is tentatively supported by Ross, Yasutake & Leek (1975) who, on the basis of their histological studies, suggested that the pneumatic duct of the air bladder might be one of the first tissues involved. However, these authors could not be certain that the air bladder was the primary site of infection.

Fish with spontaneous infections characteristically have swollen and hemorrhagic vents and the abdominal area is compressed laterally. Ross, Yasutake & Leek (1975) further noted that hemorrhaging of the caudal fin was occasionally extensive and that petechiae might occur on the lateral and ventral body surfaces. Undisturbed infected fish may swim on their side or in a vertical position with the tail down. In the terminal stages they may rest on their sides on the bottom, righting themselves when startled. The younger fry usually have a flooded air bladder whereas the older fingerlings have a watery fluid in their stomachs (Plate 24) but the air bladder is free of fluid.

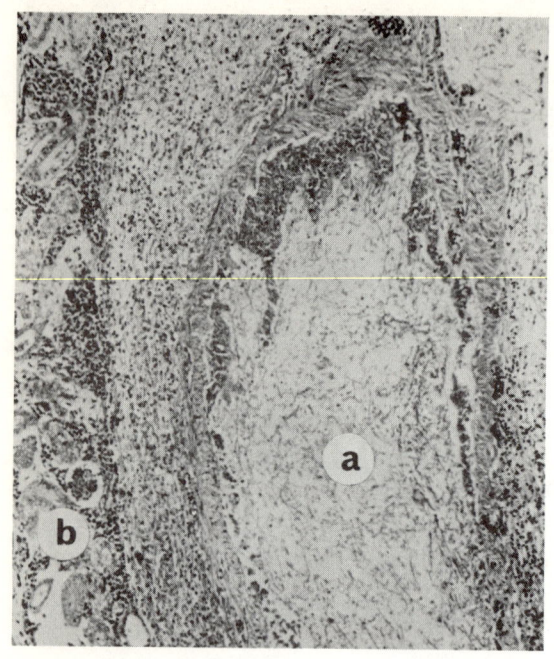

Fig. 21. *Phoma herbarum* hyphae in the air bladder (*a*) of a spring chinook salmon fry. Note inflammatory area between the kidney (*b*) and the air bladder. May-Gruenwald Giemsa stain, X 156. (Photograph courtesy of A. J. Ross, W. T. Yasutake, and S. Leek, with permission of the Journal of the Fisheries Research Board of Canada.)

Ross, Yasutake & Leek (1975) found that early in infections a small tuft of mycelium might be free in the lumen of the air bladder and can subsequently grow extensively and become systemic. These authors found that in advanced cases the entire lumen of the air bladder could become congested and hyperplasia of the bladder wall could be noted. It was also found that the fungus could penetrate the air bladder and cause an extensive inflammatory reaction in the surrounding tissues with noticeable petechiae, degeneration and necrosis of the stomach wall, kidneys, and gonads (Fig. 21; Plates 25, 26). The dorsal aorta was also congested with mycelium and hyperemic areas could be seen in the striated muscle. According to Wolke (1975), the basic inflammatory response is that of macrophage infiltration and Ross, Yasutake & Leek report that the inflammatory cells consist mainly of lymphocytes and macrophages with the histopathology being similar to that observed in coho salmon infected with *Ochroconis humicola* (Ross & Yasutake, 1973).

Wood (1974) and Ross, Yasutake & Leek (1975) have made various attempts to induce infections experimentally. The most successful attempt was made by narcotizing about 100 chinook salmon fry with M.S. 222 and then placing them in a container 2.5 to 4.0 cm deep. As the fish recovered and surfaced for air, they were exposed to a fine spray of water containing *P. herbarum* conidia. The fish were then maintained in constantly flowing water for 75 days. The first fish died thirteen days after exposure and two more twenty-six days after exposure at which time a moribund specimen was removed and found to be infected also, yielding a cumulative incidence of infection of four percent.

Some fish appear to recover spontaneously from *P. herbarum* infections. Wood (1974) found that losses usually are no longer apparent by the time the fish are 120 days old. Wood (1974) also found that examination of yearling spring chinook salmon which had the disease at 60 days of age, will reveal a few individual fish with a compact hyphal ball, about the size of a small pea, in the air bladder. These fish were presumably otherwise healthy.

Recently other *Phoma* species have been reported as parasites of vertebrates. Gordon, Salkin & Stone (1975) reported *Phoma cava* from aural dermatitis of a white-tailed deer and also *Phoma*-like pycnidia in and upon the hairs of a young child. Young, Kwon-Chung & Freeman (1973) reported a *Phoma* sp. from a subcutaneous abscess on the heel of a recipient of a renal allograft.

# ASCOMYCETES

Plehn (1916) found a septate fungus in the kidneys of two goldfish and she described this fungus as the new species *Nephromyces piscinus*, later (Plehn, 1924) changing the name to *Nephromyces piscium*. Plehn was apparently unaware of the fact that Giard (1888) had previously used the same generic name for some poorly understood fungal-like parasites found in the renal sacs of molgulid tunicates (Johnson & Sparrow, 1961). It is highly unlikely that she intended *N. piscium* to be congeneric with these organisms which it does not even remotely resemble.

Plehn (1916) was able to grow *N. piscium* in fish bouillion gelatine and on this medium the fungus produced mycelium and conidia. Using conidial suspensions pipetted into the "urethral opening" (Harnleitermündung) of two carp, Plehn was able to establish successful experimental infections.

In her discussion of the morphology of *N. piscium*, Plehn (1916) stated that she considered it to be similar to *Aspergillus* although it could not be placed in that genus.

Later, Reichenbach-Klinke (1956e) described a *Penicillium* species as a parasite of the internal organs of several freshwater fish, notably *Loricaria parva*. Reichenbach-Klinke considered this *Penicillium* species to be synonymous with *Nephromyces piscium* Plehn as well as with "fungal form a" (Reichenbach-Klinke, 1956d) and with another fungal form described by Verdun (1903). In more recent publications, he has properly adopted a more conservative stance regarding the potential synonymy of these poorly understood and inadequately described entities (Reichenbach-Klinke, 1973; Reichenbach-Klinke & Elan, 1965). In our opinion, Plehn's (1916) description and illustrations clearly show that *N. piscium* was some sort of hyphomycete but it has only the most superficial resemblance to either *Aspergillus* or *Penicillium*. We believe insufficient information is available to allow delimitation of Plehn's fungus.

There are several other problems regarding the validity of the taxon *Penicillium piscium* (Plehn) Reichenbach-Klinke, even if one accepts its highly dubious synonymy with *Nephromyces piscium*. The description of *Penicillium piscium* was based on preserved material so the organism was not cultured and cannot be compared with other *Penicillium* species. According to Reichenbach-Klinke (1956e), one of the key characteristics of *P. piscium* is its lack of a well developed ascocarp. The "ascospores" were described as ovoid, generally two-celled 4-6 X 6-10 microns brown structures. Given this description, we would question whether these were ascospores at all. Ascospores of the perfect states of other *Penicillium* species are invariably unicellular and often have a characteristic bivalve structure which causes them, in some cases, to resemble miniature pulley wheels. Our interpretation could be open to question however. Reichenbach-Klinke (1956e) used the somewhat ambiguous word "zweigeteilt" (bipartite) to describe the spores; nevertheless, from the context of his papers (1956d, e), it appears virtually certain that he intended this word to refer to septation and not to some other bilateral construction such as the bivalve structure typical of some eurotiaceous ascospores. It appears to us that the "ascospore" described by Reichenbach-Klinke (1956e) was probably some sort of chlamydospore and that he did not, in fact, observe any form of sexual reproduction in *P. piscium*. If our interpretation is correct, then Reichenbach-Klinke's comments on ascocarp development are meaningless. Also, despite Kulik's (1968) key, it must be noted that the occurrence of a *Penicillium* species as an opportunistic parasite is not sufficient grounds for designating it as a new species, especially when the observations are based on preserved material.

Taxonomic and nomenclatural problems notwithstanding, the observation of a *Penicillium* species as a parasite of a vertebrate is of interest because species of this form-genus are exceedingly common, widespread, highly adaptable moulds but are only rarely, and then often dubiously, thought to be the cause of mycotic infections of higher vertebrates (Chick, Balows & Furcolow, 1975).

# DERMOCYSTIDIUM

## INTRODUCTION

The genus *Dermocystidium* comprises a group of poorly understood, morphologically simple, protistan parasites. One of the best known species, *Dermocystidium marinum*, was long thought to be a fungus, but recent work by Perkins (1976a) has shown that it is a protozoan in the subphylum Apicomplexa and is most closely related to the coccidian Sporozoasida Leukhart. Another species, assigned to the genus *Dermocystidium* by Goldstein & Moriber (1966), lacks the relatively large well-defined, vacuoplast typical of other *Dermocystidium* species (Perkins, 1974) and is now generally thought to be synonymous with *Hyalochlorella marina*, a colorless alga related to *Chlorella* (Poyton, 1970; Perkins, 1976b).

Approximately twelve species of *Dermocystidium* have been described as parasites of fishes in freshwater in Eurasia and western North America (Pauley, 1967; Cervinka et al., 1974). These have been generally regarded as haplosporidan sporozoans (Reichenbach-Klinke & Elkan, 1965; van Duijn, 1973) or at least as some kind of sporozoan (Hoffman, 1967), but some authors have preferred to tentatively regard some species as fungi (Allen et al., 1968; Cervinka et al., 1974). The reasoning behind this is apparently based on the fact that some *Dermocystidium* species lack a lid on the spore and therefore should not be classified as haplosporidans (Allen et al., 1968). This, in turn, by process of elimination, leads to the suggestion that they might be fungi. Elkan (1962), on the other hand, considered the absence of lids on the spores of *D. gasterostei* an insufficient reason for excluding this species from the Haplosporida.

The following discussion will be limited to the *Dermocystidium* which is a parasite of Pacific salmon in western North America and to the recently described *D. cyprini*, a parasite of carp in eastern Europe. However, we hasten to add that this is done not because we are convinced that these organisms are fungi, but because they have been referred to as fungi and, as yet, there is no unequivocal evidence to show that they are not fungi. We suspect that ultimately all *Dermocystidium* species will be classified as protozoans.

## EPIZOOTIOLOGY

The *Dermocystidium* species from Pacific salmon was first described by Davis (1947) who found it on the gill filaments of an adult chinook salmon (*Oncorhynchus tshawytscha*) from the Sacramento River, California. Davis described it as a new species, *D. salmonis*, but later authors (Pauley, 1967; Allen et al., 1968) have refrained from using the specific epithet although they believed they were dealing with the same organism.

The first epizootic attributed to this organism occurred among adult chinook salmon being held in a spawning channel at the Priest Rapids Dam, Washington in November, 1965 (Pauley, 1967; Allen et al., 1968). This was followed by a similar epizootic in 1966. Prespawning mortalities in both years accounted for about 20% of the total number of fish. Fatalities among female fish were about 1.5 times greater than fatalities among male fish. Careful records kept during the 1966 epizootic showed that *Dermocystidium* cysts were present in about 77% of the unspawned carcasses. Allen et al. (1968) further noted that the *Dermocystidium* infections were not just limited to adult chinook salmon, but also occurred in emerging chinook alevins as well as coho (*Oncorhynchus kisutch*) and sockeye (*O. nerka*) salmon in the Columbia River system.

The next epizootic of which we are aware occurred among sockeye salmon in the Nimpkish River system on Vancouver Island, British Columbia during October, 1973 (G.R. Bell, pers. comm.; Hoskins, Bell & Evelyn, 1976). During this epizootic, *Dermocystidium* infections were associated with an estimated prespawning mortality of 16-22%. The exact extent to which the *Dermocystidium* infections, *per se*, were responsible for the prespawning mortalities would be difficult to determine. IHN-like virus and *Aeromonas salmonicida* were, respectively, isolated from one of five and two of five fish subjected to necropsy; nevertheless, it seems clear that the *Dermocystidium* infections were, to a large extent, responsible for the abnormally high incidence of prespawning mortalities. Wood (1974), on the other hand, suggests that bacterial gill disease following the *Dermocystidium* infection is a most important factor in precipitating the premature death of adult salmon. Cervinka et al. (1974) have noted that *D. cyprini* infections were associated with other parasitic invasions and, indeed, it would be more surprising if this were not the case.

The epizootic in the Nimpkish River system established that the incidence of serious infection by the *Dermocystidium* species from salmon was limited primarily to neither a certain species of fish (i.e., chinook salmon) nor to a specific watershed (Columbia River), but the conditions which will precipitate a serious epizootic are still unknown. The fish appear to suffer from severe infections only when the water temperature is less than 15°C but the significance of this observation is not known. Wood (1974) noted that mature cysts are readily dislodged from the gills and this lends further credence to the suggestion by Allen et al. (1968) that the source of infection might be spores shed by adults into the water; however, as yet, there is not direct evidence to support this hypothesis. It will be difficult to gain further insights into epizootiologic aspects of these infections until more is known about the life history and mode of transmission of the parasite.

## PATHOLOGY

The diagnostic features of the *Dermocystidium* species from Pacific salmon are small white cysts (Plate 27) about one mm in diameter which contain spherical cells which are usually called spores (Plates 28, 29). According to Davis (1947), the spores are about 8-10 um in diameter whereas Pauley (1967) found them to be 5-8 um in diameter. A mature spore is uninucleate and contains a large refringent vacuoplast. The cytoplasm surrounds the vacuoplast in a thin ring except at one side where it is thicker to accommodate the nucleus. The nucleus has a centrally located nucleolus ("karyosome") which is surrounded by a clear halo extending to the nuclear membrane in appropriately strained material. The cell wall of the spores is composed of coarsely granular material. The cell wall of the spores is composed of coarsely granular material with fibrillar subunits (Perkins, 1974).

Cell multiplication might occur by successive partition (Perkins, 1974), but zoosporulation has not been observed when the cells are subjected to conditions similar to the ones that induce zoosporogenesis in *D. marinum.*

In adult salmon, the rounded glistening white cysts occur primarily in the gills and oral mucosa (Plate 27). Pauley (1967) also suggested that some nonvacuolated, multinucleate cells in the spleen might represent a stage in the life history of the *Dermocystidium* species but this has not been established.

In chinook alevins, the gross pathology of the *Dermocystidium* infections is more pronounced (Allen et al., 1968). The gill coverings were usually held open by the *Dermocystidium* cysts and the hypertrophied gill tissues. The cysts could also occur in the skin, usually in the vicinity of the gills, but occasionally as far back as the caudal peduncle. There was, however, no evidence of systemic infection and both the cysts and the host reaction (fibrosis) were confined to the epithelial tissue.

Among the gill filaments of mature salmon (Pauley, 1967) the cysts are of varying size and possess a thin, clear "capsule" or "membrane" surrounding the spores. The presence of the cysts in the gill lamellae is associated with congestion and hemorrhage, lamellar fusion, lamellar epithelial hyperplasia and hypertrophy, and a mixed inflammatory response. The principal cause of death is presumably due to anoxia resulting from granulation and subacute inflammation of the gill tissue.

Attempts to culture spores from the salmon *Dermocystidium* have met with equivocal success. Allen et al. (1968) reported that they had induced the cells to grow in 1/40 thioglycollate medium resuspended in the supernatant of homogenized gill tissues to which penicillin, streptomycin and sterilized gill tissue had been added. A detailed description of the results was not given so this work is hard to evaluate.

*D. cyprini* shares several general features with the *Dermocystidium* species from salmon. It is also forms small, whitish cysts (0.6-2.0 mm in diameter) which ultimately enclose uninucleate spores, each of which contains the single refringent vacuoplast considered to be characteristic of the genus. The spores of *D. cyprini* are somewhat smaller (4-5 microns) than those of the salmon parasite and the cyst wall is somwhat thicker. Cervinka et al. (1974) have described a sequence of developmental stages for *D. cyprini* in which a small uninucleate stage develops into a large multinucleate cyst containing "plasmodia" arranged like islets in a matrix which gives an intense PAS or Grocott reaction. The plasmodia fragment into smaller plasmodia which ultimately separate into uninucleate "sporonts". The sporonts differentiate into mature spores which are released when the cyst ruptures.

## PREVENTION AND TREATMENT

Since epizootics associated with *Dermocystidium* infections appear to occur sporadically, and since the source and mode of transmission of the infections is poorly understood, methods of treatment and control are correspondingly poorly developed. Allen et al. (1968) reported that Diquat baths at a 1:500,000 dilution for one hour twice weekly appeared to provide effective prophylactic control. Chlorine and malachite green treatments appeared to be relatively ineffective.

*References
and
Index*

# References

Abbott, E.V. 1927. *Scolecobasidium*, a new genus of soil fungi. Mycologia 19: 29-31.
Agersborg, H.P.K. 1933. Salient problems in the artificial rearing of salmonid fishes, with special reference to intestinal fungisitosis and the cause of white-spot disease. Trans. Am. Fish. Soc. 63: 240-250.
Agius, C. 1978. Infection by an *Ichthyophonus*-like fungus in the deep-sea scabbard fish *Aphanopus carbo* (Lowe) (Trichiuridae) in the north east Atlantic. J. Fish Dis. 1: 191-193.
Ainsworth, G.C. 1976. An introduction to the history of mycology. Cambridge University Press, London. 359 pp.
Ajello, L. 1975. Phaeohyphomycosis: definition and etiology. Proc. Third Internat. Conference on the Mycoses, Sao Paolo, Brazil, 1974. Pan Am. Hlth. Org. Sci. Publ. 304: 126-130.
Ajello, L., M.R. McGinnis, and J. Camper. 1977. An outbreak of phaeohyphomycosis in rainbow trout caused by *Scolecobasidium humicola*. Mycopathologia 62: 15-22.
Alderman, D.J. 1976. Fungal diseases of marine animals. Pages 223-260, *in* E.B. Gareth Jones, ed., Recent advances in aquatic mycology. Paul Elek (Scientific Books) Ltd., London.
Aleem, A.A., M. Ruivo, and J. Théodoridès. 1953. Un cas de maladie à Saprolegniale chez une *Atherina* des environs des Salses. Vie Milieu 3: 44-51.
Alikunhi, K.H. 1957. Fish culture in India. Fm. Bull. Indian Coun. agric. Res. 20: 144 pp.
Allen, R.L., T.K. Meekin, G.B. Pauley, and M.P. Fujihara. 1968. Mortality among chinook salmon associated with the fungus *Dermocystidium*. J. Fish. Res. Bd Can. 25: 2467-2475.
Amlacher, E. 1965. Pathologische und histochemische Befunde bei Ichthyosporidiumbefall der Regenbogenforelle (*Salmo gairdneri*) und am "Aquarienfisch Ichthyophonus". Z. Fisch. (N.F.) 13: 85-112.
Amlacher, E. 1970. Textbook of fish diseases. T.F.H. Publications, Neptune City, New Jersey (Transl. by D.A. Conroy and R.L. Herman). 302 pp.
Apazidi, L. Kh. 1959. Razvitie griba—Vozbuditelya brankhiomikoza ryb. Veterinariya 36: 37-39.

Arasaki, S., K. Nozawa, and M. Miyake. 1958. On the pathogenetic water mold. I. Bull. Jap. Soc. scient. Fish. 23: 534-538.

Arderon, W. 1748. The substance of a letter from Mr. William Arderon F.R.S. to Mr. Henry Baker F.R.S. Phil. Trans. R. Soc. 45(487): 321-323.

Areschoug, J.E. 1844. *Achlya prolifera*, växande på lefvande fisk. Öfvers. K. VetenskAkad. Förh. 1: 124-126. (summarized in Flora 28: 59-60, 1845).

Ashley, L.M. 1972. Nutritional pathology. Pages 439-537, *in* J.E. Halver, ed., Fish Nutrition. Academic Press, New York.

Ashley, L.M., J.E. Halver, and R.R. Smith. 1975. Ascorbic acid deficiency in rainbow trout and coho salmon and effects on wound healing. Pages 769-786, *in* W.E. Ribelin and G. Migaki, eds., The pathology of fishes. University of Wisconsin Press, Madison.

Barron, G.L., and L.F. Busch. 1962. Studies on the soil hyphomycete *Scolecobasidium*. Can. J. Bot. 40: 77-84.

Barthelmes, D., T. Mattheis, and J. Meyer. 1968. Kiemenfaüle bei Regenbogenforellen. Dt. FischZtg., Radebeul 15: 296-300.

Bartsch, A. 1968. Eine andere Pilzerkrankung. Öst. Fisch. 21: 153-155.

Batista, A.C., and H. da Silva Maia. 1959. Uma nova doença fungica de peixe ornamental. Anais Soc. Biol. Pernamb. 16: 153-159.

Bauduoy, A.M., and G. Tuffery. 1973. Connaissances actuelles sur un syndrome mycosique affectant les populations piscicoles des rivières à salmonidés de la France. Bull. fr. Piscic. 249: 127-142.

Bauer, O.N., V.A. Musselius, and Y.A. Strelkov. 1973. Diseases of pond fishes. Israel Program for Scientific Translations, Jerusalem. 220 pp. (Transl. of Bolezni Prudovykh Ryb, Izdatel'stvo "Kolos," Moskva, 1969.) (Available from U.S. Dept. Commerce, NTIS, Springfield, Virginia 22151.)

Beakes, G.W., and J.L. Gay. 1977. Gametangial nuclear division and fertilization in *Saprolegnia furcata* as observed by light and electron microscopy. Trans. Brit. mycol. Soc. 69: 459-471.

Bell, G.R., and G.E. Hoskins. 1971. Investigations of wild fish mortalities in B.C., 1969-1970. Fish. Res. Bd Can., Tech. Rep. No. 245. 17 pp.

Bellet, R. 1959. L'ichthyophonaise des truites d'élevage. Coll. Trav. Path. Comp., Paris. (not seen, cited by Amlacher, 1965).

Benecke, B. 1886. The enemies of pond culture in central Europe. Bull. U.S. Fish Comm. 6 (1887): 337-342. (Transl. of Die Feinde der Teichwirtschaft from Die Teichwirtschaft, Berlin, 1885.)

Benjamin, R.K. 1962. A new *Basidiobolus* that forms microspores. Aliso 5: 223-233.

Bennet, J.H. 1842. On the parasitic vegetable structures found growing in living animals. Trans. R. Soc. Edinb. 15(1844): 277-294.

Berkeley, M.J. 1864. Egg parasites and their relatives. Intellectual Observer 5: 147-153.
Bespalyi, I.I. 1949. Brankhiomikoz karpa. Trudy Inst. ryb. Zool. Akad. Nauk Ukr. SSR, Kiev. Vol. 2. (not seen, cited by Bauer et al., 1973).
Bespalyi, I.I. 1950. Zhabernaya gnil'karpa i mery bor'by s nei. Izdatel'stvo Akad. Nauk Ukr. SSR, Kiev, (not seen, cited by Bauer et al., 1973).
Bhargava, K.S., K. Swarup and C.S. Singh. 1971. Fungi parasitic on certain fresh water fishes of Gorakhpur. Indian Biol. 3: 65-69.
Bisset, K.A. 1946. The effect of temperature on non-specific infections of fish. J. Path. Bact. 58: 251-258.
Blanc, H. 1888. Notice sur une mortalité exceptionelle des brochets du lac Léman en 1887. Bull. Soc. vaud. Sci. Nat. 23: 33-37.
Blanc, M., J. Banarescu, J.L. Gaudet, and C. Hureau. 1971. European inland water fish, a multilingual catalogue. Fishing News (Books) Ltd., London, n.p.
Blazer, V.S., and R.E. Wolke. 1978. An *Exophiala*-like fungus as the cause of a systemic mycosis of marine fish. J. Fish Dis. 2: 145-152.
Boerema, G.H. 1964. *Phoma herbarum* Westend., the type species of the form-genus *Phoma* Sacc. Persoonia 3: 9-16.
Boerema, G.H. 1970. Additional notes on *Phoma herbarum*. Persoonia 5: 15-48.
Booth, C. 1971. The genus *Fusarium*. Commonwealth Mycological Institute, Kew, Surrey, England. 237 pp.
Bootsma, R. 1973. Infections with *Saprolegnia* in pike culture (*Esox lucius* L.) Aquaculture 2: 385-394.
Brett, J.R., J.E. Shelbourn, and C.T. Shoop. 1969. Growth rate and body composition of fingerling sockeye salmon, *Oncorhynchus nerka*, in relation to temperature and ration size. J. Fish. Res. Bd Can. 26: 2363-2394.
Brown, M.E. 1966. Irish salmon disease. Atl. Salm. J., Summer 1966: 13-15.
Brown, M.E. 1968. Biological notes—The salmon disease. Salm. Trout Mag. 183: 118-120.
Brown, M.E., and V.G. Collins. 1966. Irish salmon disease—an interim report. Salm. Trout Mag. 178: 180-188.
Bruce, J., and E.O. Morris. 1973. Psychrophilic yeasts isolated from marine fish. Antonie van Leeuwenhoek 39: 331-339.
Buchwald, N.F. 1971. Adolph Hannover und seine Infektionsversuche mit *Saprolegnia*. Friesia 9: 389-391.
Bucke, D. 1972. Some histological techniques applicable to fish tissues. Symp. zool. Soc. Lond. 30: 153-189.
Buckland, F., S. Walpole, and A. Young. 1880. Report on the disease which

has recently prevailed among the salmon in the Tweed, Eden and other rivers in England and Scotland. (C-2660), H.M.S.O., London. 125 pp.

Burrows, R.E. 1949. Prophylactic treatment for control of fungus (*Saprolegnia parasitica*) on salmon eggs. Progve Fish Cult. 11: 97-103.

Calkins, C.G. 1900. *Lymphosporidium Truttae*, nov. gen., nov. sp. the cause of a recent epidemic among brook trout, *Salvelinus fontinalis*. Zool. Anz. 23: 513-520.

Carbery, J.T. 1968. Ulcerative dermal necrosis of salmonids in Ireland. Symp. zool. Soc. Lond. 24: 39-49.

Carbery, J.T., and K.L. Strickland. 1968. Ulcerative dermal necrosis (UDN). Ir. Vet. J. 22: 171-175.

Carmichael, J.W. 1966. Cerebral mycetoma of trout due to a *Phialophora*-like fungus. Sabouraudia 5: 120-123.

Caullery, M., and F. Mesnil. 1905. Sur les haplosporidies parasites de poissons marins. C. r. Séanc. Soc. Biol. 58: 640-643.

Cervinka, S., J. Vítovec, J. Lom, J. Hoska, and F. Kubů 1974. Dermocystidiosis—a gill disease of the carp due to *Dermocystidium cyprini* n. sp. J. Fish Biol. 6: 689-699.

Chaudhuri, H., P.L. Kochhar, S.S. Lotus, M.L. Banjeree, and A.H. Khan. 1947. A handbook of Indian water moulds. Part 1. Univ. Punjab Publ. Bot. 70 pp.

Chick, E.W., A. Balows, and M.L. Furcolow, eds. 1975. Opportunistic fungal infections. Proc. Second Internat. Conf. on Opportunistic Fungal Infections. (March 20-22, 1972, V.A. Hospital, Lexington, Kentucky). Charles C. Thomas, Springfield, Illinois. 359 pp.

Chidambaram K. 1942. Fungus disease of gourami (*Osphromenus goramy* Lacépède) in a pond at Madras. Curr. Sci. 11: 289-290.

Cifferi, R. 1957. Isolamento del *Basidiobolus ranarum* da feci umane. Atti. Ist. bot. Univ. Lab. crittogam. Pavia, Ser. 5, 15: 73-79.

Clark, F.W. 1874. Reproduction of a fish's tail. Am. Nat. 8: 363-364.

Cline, T.F., and G. Post. 1972. Therapy for trout eggs infected with *Saprolegnia*. Progve Fish Cult. 34: 148-151.

Clinton, G.P. 1894. Observations and experiments on *Saprolegnia* infesting fish. Bull. U.S. Fish Comm. 13: 163-172.

Coker, W.C. 1923. The Saprolegniaceae, with notes on other water molds. University of North Carolina Press, Chapel Hill. 201 pp.

Coker, W.C., and J.N. Couch. 1924. Revision of the genus *Thraustotheca* with a description of a new species. J. Elisha Mitchell scient. Soc. 40: 197-202, pl. 38.

Coker, W.C., and V.D. Matthews. 1937. Blastocladiales, Monoblepharidales, Saprolegniales. N. Am. Flora 2: 1-76.

Collins, V.G. 1970. Recent studies of bacterial pathogens of freshwater

fish. Proc. Soc. Wat. Treat. Exam. 19: 3-31.
Collins, V.G., and M.E. Brown. 1968. The salmon disease: two scientists report some preliminary results of experiments in Co. Waterford. The Field, February, p. 351.
Conant, N.F., D.T. Smith, R.D. Baker, and J.L. Callaway. 1971. Manual of clinical mycology, 3rd ed. W.B. Saunders Co., Philadelphia. 755 pp.
Cooke, R. 1977. The biology of symbiotic fungi. John Wiley and Sons, New York. 282 pp.
Cooke, M.C. 1880. Salmon disease. J.R. microsc. Soc. 3: 998.
Cox, P. 1916. Investigations of a disease of the herring (*Clupea harengus*) in the Gulf of St. Lawrence. Contrib. Can. Biol., 1914-1915: 81-85.
Cutter, V.M., Jr. 1941. Observations on certain species of *Aphanomyces*. Mycologia 33: 220-240.
Dankó, G., J. Szabó, and J. Szakolczai. 1967. Die Kiemenfäule bei Welsen (*Silurus glanis*). Zbl. Bak. ParasitKde., Abt. II, 121: 523-531.
Daniel, G. 1933a. Studies on *Ichthyophonus hoferi*, a parasitic fungus of the herring (*Clupea harengus*). I. The parasite as it is found in the herring. Am. J. Hyg. 17: 267-276.
Daniel, G. 1933b. Studies on *Ichthyophonus hoferi*, a parasitic fungus of the herring (*Clupea harengus*). II. The gross and microscopic lesions produced by the parasite. Am. J. Hyg. 17: 491-501.
Davis, H.S. 1947. Studies on the protozoan parasites of freshwater fishes. Fishery Bull. Fish Wildl. Serv. U.S. 51: 1-29, 14 pl.
Davis, H.S. 1953. Culture and diseases of game fishes. University of California Press, Berkeley. 332 pp.
Davis, H.S., and E.C. Lazar. 1941. A new fungus disease of trout. Trans. Am. Fish. Soc. 70: 264-271.
Dayal, R. 1958. Some aquatic fungi of Allahabad—a taxonomic study. Proc. natn. Acad. Sci. India, Sect. B, 28: 49-57.
Dick, M.W. 1969. Morphology and taxonomy of the Oomycetes, with special reference to the Saprolegniaceae, Leptomitaceae and Pythiaceae. I. Sexual reproduction. New Phytol. 68: 751-775.
Dick, M.W. 1972. Morphology and taxonomy of the Oomycetes, with special reference to the Saprolegniaceae, Leptomitaceae and Pythiaceae. II. Cytogenetic systems. New Phytol. 71: 1151-1159.
Dick, M.W. 1973a. Saprolegniales. Pages 113-144, *in* G.C. Ainsworth, F.K. Sparrow, and A.S. Sussman, eds., The fungi: an advanced treatise Vol 4B. Academic Press, New York.

Dick, M.W. 1973b. Leptomitales. Pages 145-158, *in* G.C. Ainsworth, F.K. Sparrow, and A.S. Sussman, eds., The fungi: an advanced treatise Vol. 4B. Academic Press, New York.
Dick, M.W., and Win-Tin. 1973. The development of cytological theory in the Oomycetes. Biol. Rev. 48: 133-158.
Domashova, A.A. 1971. O flore vodnykh Fikomitsetov nizhnego povolzh'e. (On the flora of aquatic Phycomycetes in lower Povolzh'e). Mikol. i Fitopatol. 5: 188-193.
Donaldson, E.M., and H.M. Dye. 1975. Corticosteroid concentrations in sockeye salmon (*Oncorhynchus nerka*) exposed to low concentrations of copper. J. Fish. Res. Bd Can. 32: 533-539.
Dorier, A., and C. Degrange. 1961. L'evolution de l'*Ichthyosporidium (Ichthyophonus) hoferi* (Plehn et Mulsow) chez les salmonides d'élevage (truite arc en ciel et saumon de fontaine). Trav. Lab. Hydrobiol. Piscic. Univ. Grenoble, 1960/1961: 7-44.
Doty, M.S., and D.W. Slater. 1946. A new species of *Heterosporium* pathogenic on young chinook salmon. Am. Midl. Nat. 36: 663-665.
Drechsler, C. 1955. A southern *Basidiobolus* forming many sporangia from globose and from elongated adhesive conidia. J. Wash. Acad. Sci. 45: 49-56.
Drew, G.H. 1909. Some notes on parasitic and other diseases of fish. Parasitology 2: 193-201.
Dudka, I.A. 1964. Nekotorye biologicheskie osobennosti *Saprolegnia parasitica* Coker—vozbuditelya dermatomikosa ryb. (Some specific biological features of *Saprolegnia parasitica*, the pathogen of dermatomycosis in fish). Pages 84-86, *in* Pervaya Nauchnaya konferentsiya molodykh uchenykh biologov. Akad. Nauk Ukr. SSR, Kiev.
Dudka, I.A., and A.A. Florinskaya. 1971. Novye i redkie dlya Leningradskoi oblasti vidy vodnykh gribov iz rybovodnykh prudov. (New and rare aquatic fungal species isolated from stock ponds in the Leningrad region). Mikol. i Fitopatol. 5: 431-438.
Duff, D.C.B. 1930. A physiological study of certain parasitic Saprolegniaceae. Contr. Can. Biol. Fish. 5: 195-202.
van Duijn, C. 1973. Diseases of fishes. Iliffe Books, London. 372 pp.
Dukes, T.W. 1975. Ophthalmic pathology of fishes. Pages 383-398, *in* W.E. Ribelin and G. Migaki, eds., The pathology of fishes. University of Wisconsin Press, Madison.
Dunne, L. 1970. When disease hit trout on the Test. The Field, 16 April: 678-680.
Edington, A. 1889. On the *Saprolegnia* of salmon disease and allied forms.

Rep. Fish. Bd Scotland 7: 368-382.

Egusa, S. 1963. Studies on saprolegniasis of the eel. I. The resistance of the eel to fungus infections. Bull. Jap. Soc. scient. Fish. 29: 27-36.

Egusa, S. 1965. The existence of a primary infectious disease in the so-called "fungus disease" in pond-reared eels. Bull. Jap. Soc. scient. Fish. 31: 517-526.

Egusa, S., and Y. Ohiwa. 1972. Branchiomycosis of pond-cultured eels. Fish Pathol. 7: 79-83 (in Japanese with English summary).

Egusa, S., and T. Nishikawa. 1965. Studies of a primary infectious disease in the so-called "fungus disease" of eels. Bull. Jap. Soc. scient. Fish. 31: 804-813.

Einsele, W. 1959. Kiemenfäule bei den Reinanken (Coregonen) des Obertrumersees. Öst. Fisch. 12: 91, 92.

Elkan, E. 1962. *Dermocystidium gasterostei* n. sp., a parasite of *Gasterosteus aculeatus* L. and *Gasterosteus pungitius* L. Nature, Lond. 196: 958-960.

Elkan, E., and C.M. Philpot. 1973. Mycotic infections in frogs due to a *Phialophora*-like fungus. Sarouraudia 11: 99-105.

Ellis, M.F. 1928. *Ichthyophonus hoferi*, Plehn & Mulsow, a flounder parasite new to North American waters. Proc. Trans. N.S. Inst. Sci. 17: 185-192 (1928-1929).

Elson, K.G.R. 1968. Salmon disease in Scotland. Scott. Fish. Bull. 30: 8-16.

Erickson, J.D. 1965. Report on the problem of *Ichthyosporidium* in a rainbow trout. Progve Fish Cult. 27: 179-184.

Ermin, R. 1952. Fungus associated with a granuloma in a Turkish fish, *Aphanius chantrei* Gaillard. Zoologica 37: 43-54.

Fiessiger, J. 1903. Über die Verpilzung der Fische. Öst. FischZtg 1:8-10.

Fijan, N. 1969. Systemic mycosis in channel catfish. Bull. Wildl. Dis. Ass. 5: 109-110.

Fish, F.F. 1934. A fungus disease in fishes of the Gulf of Maine. Parasitology 26: 1-16.

Forster, R.P. 1941. The present status of the systemic fungus disease in herring of the Gulf of Maine. Bull. Mt. Desert Isl. biol. Lab., 1941: 33-35.

Gardner, G.R., and G. LaRoche. 1973 Copper-induced lesions in estuarine teleosts. J. Fish. Res. Bd Can. 30: 363-368.

Gardner, M.L.G. 1974. Impaired osmoregulation in infected salmon, *Salmo salar* L.J. mar. biol. Assn. U.K. 54: 635-639.

Giard, A. 1888. Sur les *Nephromyces*, genre nouveau de champignons parasites du rein des Molgulidées. C.r. hebd. Séanc. Acad. Sci., Paris 106: 1180-1182.

Giussani, G., I. Borroni, and E. Grimaldi. 1976. Role of unionized ammonia in predisposing gill apparatus of *Alburnus alburnus alborella* to

fungal and bacterial diseases. Mem. Ist. Ital. Idrobiol. 33: 161-175.
Glagoleva, T.P., and E.M. Malikova. 1968. Effect of malachite green on the composition of blood in Baltic salmon fingerlings. Ryb. Khoz. 45: 15-18 (in Russian).
Goldie-Smith, E.K. 1952. The sporangial phase of *Pythium undulatum* Petersen. J. Elisha Mitchell scient. Soc. 68: 273-292.
Goldstein, S, and L. Moriber. 1966. Biology of a problematic marine fungus, *Dermocystidium* spec. I. Development and cytology. Arch. Mikrobiol. 53: 1-11.
Goodsir, J. 1842. On the Conferva which vegetates on the skin of the Goldfish. Ann. Mag. nat. Hist. 9: 333-337.
Gopalakrishnan, V. 1965. A report on the diseases in the trout hatcheries and farms of Kashmir. Bull. Cent. Inland Fish. Res. Inst., Barrackpore 6: 1-18.
Gopalakrishnan, V. 1968. Diseases and parasites of fishes in warm-water ponds in Asia and the Far East. Proc. FAO World Symp. Warm-water Pond Fish Culture. Fish Rep. FAO No. 44, Vol. 5: 319-343.
Gordon, M.A., I.F. Salkin, and W.B. Stone. 1975. *Phoma (Peyronellaea)* as a zoopathogen. Sabouraudia 13: 329-333.
Green, B.R., and M.W. Dick. 1972. DNA base composition and the taxonomy of the Oomycetes. Can. J. Microbiol. 18: 963-968.
Griffin, D.H. 1966. Effect of electrolytes on differentiation in *Achlya* sp. Plant Physiol. 41: 1254-1256.
Griffon, E., and A. Maublanc. 1911. Sur une maladie des poissons causée par une Saprolegniée (Notes de pathologie végétale et animale). Bull. Soc. mycol. France 27: 473-475.
Grimaldi, E. 1971. Episodi di mortalità massiva a carico delle popolazioni di Alborella *(Alburnus alborella)* dei laghi del nord-Italia, provocati da una infezione branchiale sostenuta da miceti del genere *Branchiomyces*. Riv. ital. Piscic. Ittiop. 6(1): 11-14.
Grimaldi, E., R. Peduzzi, G. Cavicchioli, G. Giussani, and E. Spreafico. 1973. Diffusa infezione branchiale da funghi attribuiti al genere *Branchiomyces* Plehn (Phycomycetes Saprolegniales) a carico dell'ittiofauna di laghi situati a nord e a sud delle Alpi. I. Epidemiologia dell'infezione da *Branchiomyces* in ambiente lacustre. Mem. Ist. ital. Idrobiol. 30: 61-80.
Grocott, R.G. 1955. Stain for fungi in tissue sections and smears using Gmori's methenamine-silver nitrate technic. Am. J. clin. Pathol. 25: 975-979.
Gustafson, P.V., and R.R. Rucker. 1956. Studies on an *Ichthyosporidium* infection in fish: transmission and host specificity. Spec. scient. Rep. U.S. Fish Wildl. Serv. 166: 1-8.
Harant, H., and P. Vernières. 1933. Tumeur abdominale et complexe para-

sitaire chez la vairon (*Phoxinus phoxinus* L.). Archs zool. exp. gén. 75: 225-266.

Hardy, A.D. 1910. Association of alga and fungus in salmon disease. Proc. R. Soc. Victoria 23 (N.S.): 27-32.

Hargens, A.R., and M. Perez. 1975. Edema in spawning salmon. J. Fish. Res. Bd Can. 32: 2538-2541.

Harrison, F.C. 1918. Examination of affected salmon, Miramichi hatchery, New Brunswick. Contr. Can. Biol. 1917-1918: 149-168.

Harz, C.O. 1906. *Achlya Hoferi*, eine neue Saprolegniacee auf lebenden Fischen. Allg. FischZtg 31: 365-368.

Hatai, K., and S. Egusa. 1975. *Candida sake* from gastro-tympanites of amago, *Oncorhynchus rhodurus*. Bull. Jap. Soc. scient. Fish. 41: 993.

Hatai, K., and S. Egusa. 1977. Studies on visceral mycosis of salmonid fry— II. Characteristics of fungi isolated from the abdominal cavity of amago salmon fry. Fish Pathol. 11: 187-193.

Hatai, K., S. Egusa, and T. Awakura. 1977. *Saprolegnia shikotsuensis* sp. nov. isolated from kokanee salmon associated with fish saprolegniasis. Fish Pathol. 12: 105-110.

Hatai, K., S. Egusa, and T. Nomura. 1977. *Saprolegnia australis* Elliott isolated from body surface lesions of rainbow trout fingerlings. Fish Pathol. 11: 201-206.

Hatai, K., S. Egusa, S. Takahashi, and K. Ooe. 1977. Study on the pathogenic fungus of mycotic granulomatosis I. Isolation and pathogenicity of the fungus from cultured-ayu infected with the disease. Fish Pathol. 12: 129-133.

Hendricks, J.D. 1972. Two new host species for the parasitic fungus *Ichthyophonus hoferi* in the northwest Atlantic. J. Fish. Res. Bd Can. 29: 1776-1777.

Henshall, J.A. 1898. Some preliminary observations concerning the artificial culture of the grayling. Proc. Am. Fish. Soc. 27: 105-111.

Herkner, H. 1961. Beitrag zur Frage der Art- und Rassenunterschiede bei der fischpathogenen Pilzgattung *Ichthyosporidium* Caullery et Mesnil, 1905. Dissertation, Universität München. (not seen, cited by Reichenbach-Klinke, 1973).

Heuschmann, O. 1935. Kiemenfäule bei Gibeln. Z. Fisch. 33: 681-692.

Hill, B.J. 1976. Ulcerative dermal necrosis. FAO Aquacult. Bull. 8: 13-14.

Ho, H.H. 1975. A selective medium for the isolation of *Saprolegnia* spp. from freshwater. Can. J. Microbiol. 21: 1126-1128.

Hodkinson, M., and A. Hunter. 1970. Growth control of *Saprolegnia* from UDN- infected Atlantic salmon *Salmo salar* L. J. Fish Biol. 3: 245-248.

Hofer, B. 1893. Eine Salmoniden-Erkrankung. Allg. FischZtg 18: 168-171. (Vol. 8 in N.S.).

Hoffman, G.L. 1967. Parasites of North American freshwater fishes. University of California Press, Berkeley. 486 pp.
Hoffman, G.L., and F.P. Meyer. 1974. Parasites of freshwater fishes, a review of their treatment and control. T.F.H. Publications, Neptune City, New Jersey. 224 pp.
Holliman, A., and R.H. Richards. 1978. The experimental pathogenesis of *Exophiala salmonis* infection in Atlantic salmon (*Salmo salar* L.). J. Fish Dis. In press.
de Hoog, G.S. 1977. *Rhinocladiella* and allied genera. Pages 1-140, *in* The black yeasts and allied hyphomycetes. Studies in Mycology 15, Centraalbureau voor Schimmelcultures, Baarn.
de Hoog, G.S., and J.A. von Arx. 1973. Revision of *Scolecobasidium* and *Pleurophragmium*. Kavaka 1: 55-60.
Hora, S., and T.V.R. Pillay. 1962. Handbook on fish culture in the Indo-Pacific region. FAO Fish. Biol. tech. Pap. No. 14. 204 pp.
Hörter, R. 1960. Fusarium als Erreger einer Hautmykose bei Karpfen. Z. ParasitKde. 20: 355-358.
Hoshina, T., and M. Ookubo. 1956. On a fungi disease of eel. J. Tokyo Univ. Fish. 42: 1-13.
Hoshina, T., T. Sano, and M. Sunayama. 1960. Studies on the saprolegniasis of eel. J. Tokyo Univ. Fish. 47: 59-79.
Hoskins, G.E., G.R. Bell, and T.P.T. Evelyn. 1976. The occurrence, distribution and significance of infectious diseases and neoplasms observed in fish in the Pacific region up to the end of 1974. Fish. Mar. Ser., Res. Dev. tech. Rep. 609. 37 pp.
Howard, K.L. 1971. Oospore types in the Saprolegniaceae. Mycologia 63: 679-686.
Howard, K.L., R. Seymour, and T.W. Johnson, Jr. 1970. Aquatic fungi of Iceland: Saprolegniaceae. J. Elisha Mitchell scient. Soc. 86: 63-79.
Huculak, F. 1958. Über Kiemenfäule der kleinen Maräne (*Coregonus albula*) *in* der Versuchsteichwirtschaft Landek der Anstalt für Teichbiologie der polnischen Akademie der Wissenschaften. Biul. Pol. Akad. Nauk., Krakow 6: 3-22.
Huet, M. 1972. Textbook of fish culture: breeding and cultivation of fish. Fishing News (Books) Ltd., Surrey, England. (transl. by H. Kahn). 436 pp.
Hughes, G.C. 1962. Seasonal periodicity of the Saprolegniaceae in the south-eastern United States. Trans. Br. mycol. Soc. 45: 519-531.
Hume Patterson, J. 1903. On the cause of salmon disease: a bacteriological investigation. Fish. Bd Scot. Salmon Fish., (Cd. 1544) H.M.S.O., Glasgow. 52 pp.
Humphrey, J.E. 1893. The Saprolegniaceae of the United States, with notes

on other species. Trans. Am. phil. Soc. (N.S.) 17: 63-148.

Hunter, R.E. 1975. Water moulds of the river Great Ouse and its tributaries. Trans. Br. mycol. Soc. 65: 101-108.

Huntsman, A.G. 1918. Report on affected salmon in the Miramichi River, New Brunswick. Contr. Can. Biol. 1917-1918: 169-173.

Huxley, T.H. 1882a. On *Saprolegnia* in relation to the salmon disease. Q. J. microsc. Soc. 22 (N.S.): 311-333. (extracted from Walpole, S. and T.H. Huxley. 1882. Report on the inspectors of salmon fisheries (England and Wales), 1881. 21st A. Rep., (C. 3217) H.M.S.O., London.) (reprinted in Bull. U.S. Fish Comm. 1(1881): 429-448. Issued in 1882.)

Huxley, T.H. 1882b. A contribution to the pathology of the epidemic known as the salmon disease. Proc. R. Soc. 33: 381-389. (also appeared in Nature, Lond. 25: 437-440, 1881/1882.)

Ivasik, V.M., and I.F. Demchenko. 1959. Brankhiomikoz karpa i mery bor'by s nim v prudovykh khozyaistvakh zapadnykh oblastei Ukrainskoi SSR. Nauchno-tekh. Byull. VNIORKh, No. 8. (not seen, cited by Bauer et al., 1973).

Jackson, G.A. 1974. A review of the literature on the use of copper sulfate in fisheries. U.S. Fish Wildl. Serv., Div. Popul. Reg. Res., Rep. No. FWS-LR-74-06. 88 pp. (Available from U.S. Dept. Commerce, NTIS, Springfield, Virginia 22151.)

Jensen, M.H. 1965. Disease among salmon in Irish rivers. Report to the Minister for Agriculture and Fisheries, Dublin. (not seen, cited by Carbery, 1968).

Jepps, M.W. 1937. On the protozoan parasites of *Calanus finmarchicus* in the Clyde Sea area. Q.J. microsc. Sci. (N.S.) 79: 589-658.

Jha, B.C., R.N. Seth, and K.P. Srivastava. 1977. Occurrence of *Achlya* sp. on a new host *Mystus* spp., a catfish. Curr. Sci. 46: 60.

Johnson, T.W., Jr. 1956. The genus *Achlya:* morphology and taxonomy. University of Michigan Press, Ann Arbor. 180 pp.

Johnson, T.W., Jr. 1974. Aquatic fungi of Iceland: biflagellate species. Acta Nat. Isl. 23: 1-40.

Johnson, T.W., Jr., and F.K. Sparrow, Jr. 1961. Fungi in oceans and estuaries. J. Cramer, Weinheim. 668 pp.

Johnston, T.H. 1917. Notes on a *Saprolegnia* epidemic amongst Queensland fish. Proc. R. Soc. Qd. 29: 125-131.

Johnstone, J. 1906. Internal parasites and diseased conditions of fishes. Proc. Trans. Lpool. biol. Soc. 20: 259-329. (1905-1906)

Johnstone, J. 1913. Diseased conditions of fishes. Proc. Trans. Lpool. biol. Soc. 27: 196-218.

Johnstone, J. 1920. On certain parasites, diseased and abnormal conditions of fishes. Lancs. Sea Fish. Lab., Rep. for 1919, No. 28, pp. 24-33.

Kahls, O. 1930. Über das Vorkommen von Algen und Pilzen bei Fischen. Z. Fisch. 28: 253-262. (not seen, cited by Reichenbach-Klinke & Elkan, 1965).

Kanouse, B.B. 1932. A physiological and morphological study of *Saprolegnia parasitica*. Mycologia 24: 431-452.

Keiz. G. 1959. Über die Kiemenfäule der Teichfische. Öst. Fisch. 12: 17-22.

Kendrick, W.B., and J.W. Carmichael. 1973. Hyphomycetes. Pages 323-509, in G.C. Ainsworth, F.K. Sparrow, and A.S. Sussman, eds., The fungi: an advanced treatise. Vol 4A. Academic Press, New York.

de Kinkelin, P., and Y. le Turdu. 1971. L'enzootie d' "ulcerative dermal necrosis" du saumon (*Salmo salar* L. 1766) en Bretagne. Bull. fr. Piscic. 241: 115-126.

Kirilenko, T.S., and M.A. All-Achmed. 1977. *Ochroconis tshawytschae* (Doty & Slater) comb. nov. Mikrobiol. Zh. 39: 303-306.

Kokhanskaya, Y.M. 1973. The effect of ultraviolet radiation on the eggs of the sevryuga (*Acipenser stellatus* (Pallas)). J. Ichthyol. 13: 406-413.

Krampitz, L.O., and D.W. Woolley. 1944. The manner of inactivation of thiamine by fish tissue. J. biol. Chem. 152: 9-17.

Krause, R. 1960. Untersuchungen über den Einfluß der Außenfaktoren auf die Bildung der Oogonien bei *Saprolegnia ferax* (Gruith.) Thuret. Arch. Microbiol. 36: 373-386.

Kreger-van Rij, N.J.W. 1973. Endomycetales, basidiomycetous yeasts and related fungi. Pages 11-32, in G.C. Ainsworth, F.K. Sparrow, and A.S. Sussman, eds., The fungi: an advanced treatise. Vol. 4A. Academic Press, New York.

Kulik, M. M. 1968. A compilation of descriptions of new *Penicillium* species. Agric. Handb. agric. Res. Serv., U.S.D.A. No. 351, U.S. Govt. Print. Off., Washington. 80 pp.

Kwon-Chung, K.J. 1976. Morphogenesis of *Filobasidiella neoformans*, the sexual state of *Cryptococcus neoformans*. Mycologia 68: 821-833.

Lam, T.J. 1972. Prolactin and hydromineral regulation in fishes. Gen. comp. Endocr. Suppl. 3: 328-338.

Landolt, M.L. 1975. Visceral granuloma and nephrocalcinosis of trout. Pages 793-801, in W.E. Ribelin and G. Migaki, eds., The pathology of fishes. University of Wisconsin Press, Madison.

Laveran, A., and A. Pettit. 1910. Sur un épizootie des truites. C. r. hebd. Séanc. Acad. Sci., Paris 151: 421-423.

Lee, P.C., Jr. 1962. Some effects of pH, temperature and light on the production of zoosporangia in *Saprolegnia parasitica* Coker. M.A. Thesis, University of Richmond, Virginia. 36 pp.

Lee, P.C., Jr., and W.W. Scott. 1967. Effects of light and temperature on the formation of sexual structures in the family Saprolegniaceae. Res. Div., Virginia Polytech. Inst., Bull. 2, Biol. Dept., 35 pp.

Léger, L. 1924. Sur un organisme du type Ichthyophone parasite du tube digestif de la Lote d'eau douce. C. r. hebd. Séanc. Acad. Sci., Paris 197: 785-787.

Léger, L. 1927. Sur la nature et l'évolution des "sphérules" décrites chez les Ichthyophones, Phycomycètes parasites de la Truite. C. r. hebd. Séanc. Acad. Sci., Paris 184: 1268-1271.

Léger, L., and E. Hesse. 1923. Sur un champignon du type *Ichthyophonus* parasite de l'intestin de la Truite. C. r. hebd. Séanc. Acad. Sci., Paris 176: 420-422.

Lennon, R.E. 1954. Feeding mechanism of the sea lamprey and its effect on host fishes. Fish. Bull. Fish Wildl. Serv. U.S. 56: 247-293.

Lopukhina, A.M. 1959. Zabolevaniya sigovykh i amurskikh ryb pri ikh sovmestnon vyrashchivanii v prudovykh khozyaistvakh USSR. Trudy Soveshch., Ikhtiol. Kom. Akad. Nauk. SSSR, No. 9: 110-113.

Lucký, Z. 1970. The occurrence of branchiomycosis in the *Silurus glanis*. Acta vet. Brno 39: 187-192.

Machado-Cruz, J.A. 1961. Nouveau hôte d'*Ichthyosporidium (Gadus morhua* L.). Bolm Soc. port. Ciênc. nat., 2 sér., 8: 212-215.

Maurizio, A. 1895. Die Pilzkrankheit der Fische und der Fischeier. Z. Fisch. 4: 76-89. (Reprinted in Mitt dt. FischVer 3: 1-14.)

Maurizio, A. 1896. Studien über Saprolegnieen. Flora 82: 14-31.

Maurizio, A. 1897a. Die Pilzkrankheit der Fische und der Fischeier. Zentbl. Bakt. ParasitKde. 22: 408-410.

Maurizio, A. 1897b. Les maladies causées aux poissons et aux oeufs de poissons par les champignons. Rev. mycologique 19: 77-85.

Maurizio, A. 1899. Beitrage zür Biologie der Saprolegnieen. Mitt. dt. FischVer. 7: 1-66.

Mazilkin, I.A. 1957. Biologicheskii metod borby s saprolegniei. Proc. Conference on Fisheries, Moscow, 1954: 81-87.

McGinnis, M.R. 1977. *Exophiala spinifera*, a new combination for *Phialophora spinifera*. Mycotaxon 5: 337-340.

McGinnis, M.R., and L. Ajello. 1974a. A new species of *Exophiala* isolated from channel catfish. Mycologia 66: 518-520.

McGinnis, M.R., and L. Ajello. 1974b. *Scolecobasidium tshawytschae*. Trans. Br. mycol. Soc. 63: 202-203.

McGinnis, M.R., and L. Ajello. 1975. *Scolecobasidium macrosporum* as a synonym of *Scolecobasidium tshawytschae*. Mycotaxon 2: 132-134.

McGinnis, M.R., and A.A. Padhye. 1977. *Exophiala jeanselmei*, a new combination for *Phialophora jeanselmei*. Mycotaxon 5: 341-352.

McKay, D.L. 1967. *Saprolegnia diclina* Humphrey as a parasite of the salmonid, *Oncorhynchus kisutch*. M. Sc. Thesis, University of British Columbia, Vancouver. 63 pp.

McLeay, D.J. 1975. Variations in the pituitary-interrenal axis and the abundance of circulating blood-cell types in juvenile coho salmon, *Oncorhynchus kisutch*, during stream residence. Can. J. Zool. 53: 1882-1891.

McVicar, A.H., and K. MacKenzie. 1972. A fungus disease of fish. Scott. Fish. Bull. 37: 27-28.

Meier, A.H. 1972. Temporal synergism of prolactin and adrenal steroids. Gen. comp. Endocr. Suppl. 3: 499-508.

Meier, W., K. Klinger, and R. Müller. 1977. Ulzerative Dermalnekrose (UDN) der Bachforelle (*Salmo trutta fario*) in der Schweiz. Teil II: Prädisponierende und infektionsbegünstigende Faktoren. Schweizer Arch. Tierheilk. 119: 277-291.

Meier, W., K. Klinger, R. Müller, and H. Luginbühl. 1977. Ulzerative Dermalnekrose (UDN) der Bachforelle (*Salmo trutta fario*) in der Schweiz. Teil I: Makroskopische und mikroskopische Befunde. Schweizer Arch. Tierheilk. 119: 235-245.

Meuron, P.-A. de, and H. Burgisser. 1973. A propos du diagnostic des maladies chez les poissons. Schweizer Arch. Tierheilk. 115: 184-189.

Meyer, F.P., and J.A. Robinson. 1973. Branchiomycosis: a new fungal disease of North American fishes. Progve Fish Cult. 35: 74-77.

Miyazaki, T., and S. Egusa. 1972. Studies on mycotic granulomatosis in freshwater fishes—I. The goldfish. Fish Pathol. 7: 15-25 (in Japanese).

Miyazaki, T., and S. Egusa. 1973a. Studies on mycotic granulomatosis in freshwater fishes—II. Ayu, *Plecoglossus altivelis*. Fish Pathol. 7: 125-133. (in Japanese).

Miyazaki, T., and S. Egusa. 1973b. Studies on mycotic granulomatosis in freshwater fishes—III. Blue gill. Fish Pathol. 8: 41-43. (in Japanese).

Miyazaki, T., and S. Egusa. 1973c. Studies on mycotic granulomatosis in freshwater fishes-IV. Wild fishes. Fish Pathol. 8: 44-47. (in Japanese).

Miyazaki, T., S. Kubota, and F. Tashiro. 1977. Studies on visceral mycosis of salmonid fry—I. Histopathology. Fish Pathol. 11: 183-186.

Möller, H. 1974. *Ichthyosporidium hoferi* (Plehn et Mulsow) (Fungi) as parasite in the Baltic cod (*Gadus morhua* L.). Kieler Meeresforsch. 30: 37-41.

Monsma, E.Y. 1937. A study of the water molds of the Lydell State Fish Hatchery at Comstock Park, Michigan. Pap. Michigan Acad. Sci. 22: 165-182.

Montpellier, J., and R. Dieuzeide. 1933. Pseudo-tumeur mycélienne chez un poisson (*Cyprinodon fasciatus* Val.). Bull. Trav. Stn. Agric. Pêche Castiglione (1932) 1: 551-557.

Munro, A.L.S. 1970. Ulcerative dermal necrosis, a disease of migratory salmonid fishes in the rivers of the British Isles. Biol. Conserv. 2: 129-132.

Murphy, T. 1973. Ulcerative dermal necrosis (UDN) of salmonids—a review. Ir. vet. J. 27: 85-90.

Neish, G.A. 1975a. Observations on the growth and morphology of Emerson's *Saprolegnia* sp. 47-15a. Can. J. Bot. 53: 1423-1427.

Neish, G.A. 1975b. Carbenicillin as an aid in obtaining bacteria-free cultures of *Saprolegnia* species. Mycologia 67: 1192-1197.

Neish, G.A. 1976. Observations on the pathology of saprolegniasis of Pacific salmon and on the identity of the fungi associated with this disease. Ph.D. Thesis, University of British Columbia, Vancouver. 213 pp.

Neish, G.A. 1977. Observations on saprolegniasis of adult sockeye salmon, *Oncorhynchus nerka* (Walbaum). J. Fish Biol. 10: 513-522.

Neish, G.A., and B.R. Green. 1976. Nuclear and satellite DNA base composition and the taxonomy of *Saprolegnia* (Oomycetes). J. gen. Microbiol. 96: 215-219.

Nelson, N.C. 1974. A review of the literature on the use of malachite green in fisheries. Fish Wildl. Serv. U.S., Div. Popul. Reg. Res., Rep. No. FWS-LR-74-11. 79 pp. (Available from U.S. Dept. Commercer, NTIS, Springfield, Va. 22151). 79 pp.

Neresheimer, E., and C. Clodi. 1914. *Ichthyophonus hoferi* Plehn u. Mulsow, der Erreger der Taumelkrankheit der Salmoniden. Arch. Protistenk. 34: 217-248.

Nickerson, M.A., and J.A. Hutchison. 1971. The distribution of the fungus *Basidiobolus ranarum* Eidam in fish, amphibians and reptiles. Am. Midl. Nat. 86: 500-502.

Nigrelli, R.F. 1946. Studies on the marine resources of southern New England. V. Parasites and diseases of the oceanpout, *Macrozoarces americanus*. Bull. Bingham Oceanogr. Coll. 9: 187-221.

Nolard-Tintigner, N. 1970. Deux épidémies de saprolégniose des poissons par *Saprolegnia ferax* (Gruith.) et par *Saprolegnia diclina* (Humphrey). Annls Parasit. hum. comp. 45: 761-770.

Nolard-Tintigner, N. 1971. Cause de la mort dans la saprolégniose expérimentale du poisson. Bull. Acad. r. Belg. Cl. Sci. 57: 185-191.

Nolard-Tintigner, N. 1973. Etude expérimentale sur l'épidémiologie et la pathogenie de la saprolégniose chez *Lebistes reticulatus* Peters et *Xiphophorus helleri* Heckel. Acta zool. path. Antverp. 57: 1-127.

Nolard-Tintigner, N. 1974. Contribution à l'étude de la Saprolégniose des poissons en région tropicale. Acad. r. Sci. outre-mer, Cl. Sci. nat. méd. (N.S.) 19: 1-58.

O'Bier, A.H., Jr. 1960. A study of the aquatic Phycomycetes associated with diseased fish and fish eggs. Ph.D. Thesis, Virginia Polytechnic Institute, Blacksburg. 77 pp.

O'Brien, D.J. 1974. Use of lesion filtrates for transmission of UDN (ulcerative dermal necrosis) in salmonids. J. Fish Biol. 6: 507-511.

Olivereau, M. 1962. Modifications de l'interrénal du smolt (*Salmo salar* L.) au cours du passage d'eau douce en eau de mer. Gen. comp. Endocr. 2: 565-573.

Oseid, D.M. 1977. Control of fungus growth on fish eggs by *Asellus militaris* and *Gammarus pseudolimnaeus*. Trans. Am. Fish. Soc. 106: 192-195.

Otte, E. 1964. Eine Mykose bei einem Stachelrochen (*Trigon pastinacae* L.). Wien. tierärztl. Mschr. 51: 171-175.

Pauley, G.B. 1967. Prespawning adult salmon mortality associated with a fungus of the genus *Dermocystidium*. J. Fish. Res. Bd Can. 24: 843-848.

Peduzzi, R. 1973. Diffusa infezione branchiale da funghi attribuiti al genere *Branchiomyces* Plehn (Phycomycetes Saprolegniales) a carico dell'ittiofauna di laghi situati a nord e a sud delle Alpi. II. Esigenze colturali, trasmissione sperimentale ed affinità tassonomiche del micete. Mem. Ist. ital. Idrobiol. 30: 81-96.

Peduzzi, R., and S. Bizzozero. 1977. Immunological investigation of four *Saprolegnia* species with parasitic activity in fish: serological and kinetic characterization of a chymotrypsin-like activity. Microb. Ecol. 3: 107-118.

Peduzzi, R.,N. Nolard-Tintigner, and S. Bizzozero. 1976. Recherches sur la saprolégniose. II. Etude du processus de pénétration, mise en évidence d'une enzyme protéolytique et aspect histopathologique. Riv. ital. Piscic. Ittiop. 11: 109-117.

Perkins, F.O. 1974. Phylogenetic considerations of the problematic thraustochytriaceous-labrynthulid-*Dermocystidium* complex based on observations of fine structure. Veröff Inst. Meeresforsch. Bremerh., Suppl. 5: 45-63.

Perkins, F.O. 1976a. Zoospores of the oyster pathogen, *Dermocystidium marinum*. 1. Fine structure of the conoid and other sporozoan-like organelles. J. Parasit. 62: 959-974.

Perkins, F.O. 1976b. Fine structure of lower marine and estuarine fungi. Pages 279-312, *in* E.B. Gareth Jones, ed., Recent advances in aquatic mycology. Paul Elek (Scientific Books) Ltd., London.

Pettit, A. 1911. A propos du microorganisme producteur de la Taumelkrankheit: *Ichthyosporidium* ou *Ichthyophonus*. C.r. Séanc. Soc. Biol., Paris 70: 1045-1047.

Pettit, A. 1913. Observations sur l'*Ichthyosporidium* et sur la maladie qu'il provoque chez la truite. Annls Inst. Pasteur, Paris 27: 986-1008.

Pickering, A.D., and L.G. Willoughby. 1977. Epidermal lesions and fungal infection on the perch, *Perca fluviatilis* L., in Windermere. J. Fish Biol. 11: 349-354.

Pierotti, P. 1971. Su di un particolare episodio di micosi in *Tinca tinca*. Atti Soc. ital. Sci. vet. 25: 361-363.

Plehn, M. 1912. Eine neue Karpfenkrankheit und ihr Erreger: *Branchiomyces sanguinis*. Zentbl. Bakt. ParasitKde., Abt. 1, Orig. Bd., 62: 129-134.

Plehn, M. 1916. Pathogene Schimmelpilze in der Fischniere. Z. Fisch. 18: 51-54.

Plehn, M. 1924. Praktikum der Fischkrankheiten. E. Schweitzerbart'sche Verlags Stuttgart. 179 pp.

Plehn, M., and K. Mulsow. 1911. Der Erreger der "Taumelkrankheit" der Salmoniden. Zentbl. Bakt. ParasitKde., Abt. 1, 58: 63-68.

Powles, P.M., D.G. Garnett, G.D. Ruggieri, and R.F. Nigrelli. 1968. *Ichthyophonus* infection in yellowtail flounder (*Limanda ferruginea*) off Nova Scotia. J. Fish. Res. Bd Can. 25: 597-598.

Poyton, R.O. 1970. The characterization of *Hyalochlorella marina* gen. et sp. nov. a new colorless counterpart of *Chlorella*. J. gen. Microbiol. 62: 171-188.

Priebe, K. 1973. Nekrosebezirk in der Körpermuskulatur eines Köhlers (*Pollachius virens*) mit Befall von *Ichthyosporidium hoferi*. Dt. tierärztl. Wschr. 80: 197-220.

Pyefinch, K.A., and K.G.R. Elson. 1967. Salmon disease in Irish rivers. Scott. Fish. Bull. 26: 1-4.

Raciborski, M. 1886. Roslinne pasorzyty karpi. (Vegetative parasites of carp). Rozpr. Akad. Umiejet., Ser. 1, 14: 149-168.

Radulescu, J., N. Vasiliu-Suceveanu, and S. Luscan. 1957. Infestatie accidentala la coregon. Bul. Inst. Cerc. pisc. Anul. 16(3). (not seen, cited by Bauer et al., 1973).

Ramsbottom, J. 1916. Some notes on the history of the classification of the Phycomycetes. Trans. Br. mycol. Soc. 5: 324-350.

Rehulka, J., and J. Tesarcik. 1972. Findings of branchiomycoses during diagnostical work of the group for diseases and protection of fish in the Czechoslovak Agricultural Academy, Research Institute for Pisciculture and Hydrobiology in Vodnany in the years 1961-1970. Acta. vet. Brno 41: 101-106.

Reichenbach-Klinke, H.-H. 1954. Untersuchungen über die bei Fischen durch Parasiten hervorgerufenen Zysten und deren Wirkung auf den Wirtskörper. I.Z. Fisch. (N.S.) 3: 565-636.

Reichenbach-Klinke, H.-H. 1955. Pages 351-357, *in* Pilze in Tumoren bei Fischen. Zool. Anz. Suppl., Verh. dt. zool. Ges. Tübingen 1954. Leipzig.

Reichenbach-Klinke, H.-H. 1956a. Die Vermehrungsformen des zoophagen Pilzes *Ichthyosporidium hoferi* (Plehn et Mulsow) (Fungi, Phycomycetes) im Wirt. Veröff. Inst. Meeresforsch. Bremerh. 4: 214-219.

Reichenbach-Klinke, H.-H. 1956b. Augenschäden bei Meeresfischen durch den Pilz *Ichthyosporidium hoferi* (Plehn et Muslow) und Bemerkungen zu seiner Verbreitung bei Mittelmeerfischen. Pubbl. Stn. zool. Napoli 29: 22-32.
Reichenbach-Klinke, H.-H. 1956c. Verbreitung und Bekämpfung des Pilzes *Ichthyosporidium hoferi* (Plehn et Mulsow) (= *Ichthyophonus hoferi*). Aquar.-u. Terrar.-Z. (DATZ) 9: 70-72.
Reichenbach-Klinke, H.-H. 1956d. Über einige bisher unbekannte Hyphomyceten bei verschiedenen Süsswasser-und Meeresfischen. Mycopathol. Mycol. appl. 7: 333-347.
Reichenbach-Klinke, H.-H. 1956e. Eine Aspergillacee (Fungi, Ascomycetes, Plectascales) als Endoparasit bei Süsswasserfischen. Veröff. Inst. Meeresforsch. Bremerh. 4: 111-116.
Reichenbach-Klinke, H.-H. 1960. Die Discus-Krankheit und ihre Ursachen. Aquar.-u. Terrar.-Z. (DATZ) 13: 303-305.
Reichenbach-Klinke, H.-H. 1973. Reichenbach-Klinke's fish pathology (with collaboration by M. Landolt). T.F.H. Publications, Neptune City, New Jersey. 512 pp. (Transl. of Krankheiten und Schädigungen der Fische. Gustav Fischer Verlag, Stuttgart, 389 pp., 1966.)
Reichenbach-Klinke, H.-H. 1974. Die Erscheinungsformen der UDN (Ulcerative Dermalnekrose)., in Die Furunkulose und neuere Infektionskrankheiten der Süsswasserfische. Münchn. Beitr. Abwass.-Fisch.-Flussbiol. 25: 47-54.
Reichenbach-Klinke, H.-H. 1975. Lesions due to drugs. Pages 647-656, *in* W.E. Ribelin and G. Migaki, eds., The pathology of fishes. University of Wisconsin Press, Madison.
Reichenbach-Klinke, H.-H., and E. Elkan. 1965. The principal diseases of lower vertebrates. Academic Press, New York. 600 pp.
Reichle, G. 1973. Beobachtungen zur Kiemenfäule beim Karpfen. Öst. Fisch. 26: 58, 59.
Richards, R.H., and A.D. Pickering. 1978. Frequency and distribution patterns of *Saprolegnia* infection in wild and hatchery-reared brown trout *Salmo trutta* L. and char *Salvelinus alpinus* (L.). J. Fish Dis. 1: 69-82.
Richards, R.H., A. Holliman, and S. Helgason. 1978. Naturally occurring *Exophiala salmonis* infection in Atlantic salmon (*Salmo salar* L.). J. Fish Dis. 1: 357-369.
Roberts, R.E. 1963. A study of the distribution of certain numbers of the Saprolegniaceae. Trans. Br. mycol. Soc. 46: 213-224.
Roberts, R.J. 1972. Ulcerative dermal necrosis (UDN) of salmon (*Salmo salar* L.). Symp. zool. Soc. Lond. 30: 53-81.
Roberts, R.J., and C.J. Shepherd. 1974. Handbook of trout and salmon

diseases. Fishing News (Books) Ltd., Surrey, England. 168 pp.
Roberts, R.J., W.M. Shearer, A.L.S. Munro, and K.G.R. Elson. 1969. The pathology of ulcerative dermal necrosis of Scottish salmon. J. Path. 97: 563-565.
Roberts, R.J., H.J. Ball, A.L.S. Munro, and W.M. Shearer. 1971. Studies on ulcerative dermal necrosis of salmonids III. The healing process in fish maintained under experimental conditions. J. Fish Biol. 3: 221-224.
Roberts, R.J., A. McQueen, W.M. Shearer, and H. Young. 1973. The histopathology of salmon tagging III. Secondary infections associated with tagging. J. Fish Biol. 5: 621-623.
Roberts, R.J., W.M. Shearer, A.L.S. Munro, and K.G.R. Elson. 1970. Studies on ulcerative dermal necrosis of salmonids II. The sequential pathology of the lesions. J. Fish Biol. 2: 373-378.
Robertson, M. 1908. Notes upon a Haplosporidian belonging to the genus *Ichthyosporidium*. Proc. R. Phys. Soc. Edinb. (1906-1909) 17: 175-187.
Robertson, M. 1909. Notes on an Ichthyosporidian causing a fatal disease in sea-trout. Proc. zool. Soc. Lond., 1909: 399-402.
Robertson, O.H., S. Hane, B.C. Wexler, and A.P. Rinfret. 1963. The effect of hydrocortisone on immature rainbow trout (*Salmo gairdneri*). Gen. comp. Endocr. 3: 422-436.
Robin, C. 1853. Histoire naturelle des végétaux parasites qui croissent sur l'homme et sur les animaux vivants. J.-B. Baillière, Paris, 702 pp.
Roddie, J.C., and W.F.M. Wallace. 1975. The physiology of disease. Lloyd-Luke (Medical Books) Ltd., London. 588 pp.
Ross, A.J., and T.J. Parisot. 1958. Record of the fungus *Ichthyosporidium* Caullery and Mesnil, 1905, in Idaho. J. Parasit. 44: 453-454.
Ross, A.J., and W.T. Yasutake. 1973. *Scolecobasidium humicola*, a fungal pathogen of fish. J. Fish. Res. Bd Can. 30: 994-995.
Ross, A.J., W.T. Yasutake, and S. Leek. 1975. *Phoma herbarum*, a fungal plant saprophyte as a fish pathogen. J. Fish. Res. Bd Can. 32: 1648-1652.
Roth, R.R. 1972. Some factors contributing to the development of fungus infections in freshwater fish. J. Wildl. Dis. 8: 24-28.
Roy, R.Y., R.S. Dwivedi, and R.R. Mishra. 1962. Two new species of *Scolecobasidium* from soil. Lloydia 25: 164-166.
Rucker, R.R. 1944. A study of *Saprolegnia* infections among fish. Ph.D. Thesis, University of Washington, Seattle. 92 pp.
Rucker, R.R. 1963. Formalin in the hatchery. Progve Fish Cult. 25: 203-207.
Rucker, R.R., and P.V. Gustafson. 1953. An epizootic among rainbow trout. Progve Fish Cult. 15: 179-181.
Ruggieri, G.D., R.F. Nigrelli, P.M. Powles, and D.G. Garnett. 1970. Epi-

zootics in yellowtail flounder, *Limanda ferruginea* Storer, in the western North Atlantic caused by *Ichthyophonus,* an ubiquitous parasitic fungus. Zoologica, N.Y. 55: 57-62.

Rushton, W. 1925. Biological notes. Fungus and fish. Salm. Trout Mag. No. 40: 223-258.

Rutherford, J. 1881. Observations on the salmon disease. Trans. J. Proc. Dumfries. Galloway nat. Hist. Antiq. Soc. 1881: 72-76.

Ryder, J.A. 1881. On the retardation of the development of the ova of the shad (*Alosa sapidissima*), with observations on the egg-fungus and bacteria. Bull. U.S. Fish Comm. 1: 177-190.

Ryder, J.A. 1883. Experiments with carbolic acid to kill the fungus on large fishes. Bull. U.S. Fish Comm. 2(1882): 190-191.

Salvin, S.B. 1941. Comparative studies on the primary and secondary zoospores of the Saprolegniaceae. I. Influence of temperature. Mycologia 33: 592-600.

Sandholzer, L.A., T. Nostrand, and L. Young. 1945. Studies of an Ichthyosporidian-like parasite of oceanpout (*Zoarces anguillaris*). Spec. scient. Rep. U.S. Fish Wildl. Serv. 31: 1-12.

Sarig, S. 1971. The prevention and treatment of diseases of warmwater fishes under subtropical conditions, with special emphasis on intensive fish farming. Book 3 *in* S.F. Snieszko and H.R. Axelrod, eds., Diseases of fishes. T.F.H. Publications, Neptune City, New Jersey. 127 pp.

Scattergood, L.W. 1948. A report on the appearance of the fungus *Ichthyosporidium hoferi* in the herring of the northwestern Atlantic. Spec. scient. Rep. U.S. Fish Wildl. Serv. 58: 1-33.

Scerban, N.P. 1954. Novye svedenii o zabolevanii ryby brankhiomikozom. Ryb. Khoz. 30: 54.

Schäperclaus, W. 1929. Untersuchungen über die Kiemenfäule bei Fischen. I. Beiträge zur Kenntnis der Kiemenfäule des Karpfens. Z. Fisch. 27: 271-286.

Schäpercalus, W. 1953. Fortpflanzung und Systematik von *Ichthyophonus*. Aquar.-u. Terrar.-Z. 6: 177-182.

Schäperclaus, W. 1954. Fischkrankheiten. Akademie-Verlag, Berlin. 708 pp.

Scheuring, L., and O. Gaschott. 1928. Neue Beobachtungen über die Kiemenfäule der Karpfen. Fischereizeitung 31: 475.

Scheuring, L., and E. Walter. 1926. Beobachtungen über die Kiemenfäule der Karpfen. Fischereizeitung 29: 777.

Schmitt, J.A., and E.S. Beneke. 1962. Aquatic fungi from South Bass and neighboring islands in western Lake Erie. II. Additional biflagellate and uniflagellate Phycomycetes. Ohio J. Sci. 62: 11-12.

Schnetzler, J.B. 1887. Infection d'une larve de grenouille par *Saprolegnia ferax*. Archs Sci. phys. nat., Ser. 3, 18: 492.

Schnick, R.A. 1973. Formalin as a therapeutant in fish culture. U.S. Fish Wildl. Serv., Div. Popul. Regul. Res., Rep. No. FWS-LR-74-09. 129 pp. (Available from U.S. Dept. Commerce, NTIS Spring Field, Va. 22151).

Schwartz, F.J. 1963. A new *Ichthyosporidium* parasite of the spot (*Leiostomus xanthurus*): a possible answer to the recent oyster mortalities. Progve Fish Cult. 25: 181-186.

Scott, W.W. 1956. A new species of *Aphanomyces*, and its significance in the taxonomy of the watermolds. Va J. Sci. 7 (N.S.): 170-175.

Scott, W.W., and A.H. O'Bier, Jr. 1962. Aquatic fungi associated with diseased fish and fish eggs. Progve Fish Cult. 24: 3-15.

Scott, W.W., and C.O. Warren. 1964. Studies of the host range and chemical control of fungi associated with diseased tropical fish. Va agric. exp. Stn., Blacksburg. Tech. Bull. 171. 24 pp.

Selye, H. 1950. Stress and the general adaptation syndrome. Br. med. J. 1: 1383-1392.

Seymour, R. 1970. The genus *Saprolegnia*. Nova Hedwigia 19: 1-124.

Shanor, L., and H.B. Saslow. 1944. *Aphanomyces* as a fish parasite. Mycologia 36: 413-415.

Shcherbina, A.K. 1952. Bolezni Prudovykh Ryb. Gosudarstvennoe Izdatel' stvo Sel'skokhozyaystvennoy Literatury, Moskva. 206 pp.

Shcherbina, A.K. 1960. Bolezni Ryb i Mery Bor'by s Nimi. Izdatel'stvo Ukrainskoy Akad. Sel'skokhyaystvenykh Nauk, Kiev. 334 pp.

Shereshevskaya, E.G. 1932. Zabolevanie ryb i ryb'ey ikry saprolegniey. (Diseases of fish and fish eggs caused by *Saprolegnia*.) Ryb. Khoz. Karel. 1: 117-132.

Sills, J.B. 1974. A review of the use of lime ($Ca(OH)_2$, $CaO$, $CaCo_3$) in fisheries. U.S. Fish Wildl. Serv., Div. Popul. Reg. Res. Rep. No. FWS-LR-74-10. 30 pp. (Available from U.S. Dept. Commerce, NTIS, Springfield, Va. 22151).

Sindermann, C.J. 1956. Diseases of fishes of the western North Atlantic IV. Fungus disease and resultant mortalities of herring in the Gulf of Saint Lawrence in 1955. Res. Bull. Dep. Sea Shore Fish. Me 25: 1-23.

Sindermann, C.J. 1958. An epizootic in Gulf of Saint Lawrence fishes. Trans. N. Am. Wildl. Conf. 23: 349-360.

Sindermann, C.J. 1963. Diseases in marine populations. Trans. N. Am. Wildl. Conf. 28: 336-356.

Sindermann, C.J. 1966. Diseases of marine fishes. Adv. mar. Biol. 4: 1-89.

Sindermann, C.J. 1970. Principle diseases of marine fish and shellfish. Academic Press, New York. 369 pp.

Sindermann, C.J., and L.W. Scattergood. 1954. Diseases of fishes of the western North Atlantic. II. *Ichthyosporidium* disease of the sea herring (*Clupea harengus*). Res. Bull. Dep. Sea Shore Fish. Me 19: 1-40.

Smith, H.H. 1912. Some of the diseases affecting the Salmonidae and other fish. Salm. Trout Mag. 4: 41-48.

Snieszko, S.F. 1972. Nutritional fish diseases. Pages 403-437, *in* J.E. Halver, ed., Fish nutrition. Academic Press, New York.

Snieszko, S.F. 1974. The effects of environmental stress on outbreaks of infectious diseases of fish. J. Fish. Biol. 6: 197-208.

Sparrow, F.K., Jr. 1952. Phycomycetes from the Douglas Lake region of northern Michigan. Mycologia 44: 759-772.

Sparrow, F.K., Jr. 1973. Lagenidiales. Pages 159-163, *in* G.C. Ainsworth, F.K. Sparrow, and A.S. Sussman, eds., The fungi: an advanced treatise. Vol. 4B. Academic Press, New York.

Sprague, V. 1965. *Ichthyosporidium* Caullery and Mesnil, 1905, the name of a genus of fungi or a genus of sporozoans? Syst. Zool. 14: 110-114.

Sprague, V. 1966. *Ichthyosporidium* sp. Schwartz, 1963, parasite of the fish *Leiostomus xanthurus*, is a microsporidian. J. Protozool. 13: 356-358.

Sproston, N.G. 1944. *Ichthyosporidium hoferi* (Plehn & Mulsow, 1911), an internal fungoid parasite of the mackerel. J. mar. biol. Assn., U.K. 26: 72-98.

Srinivasan, M., and M. Thirumalachar. 1967. Studies on *Basidiobolus* species from India with discussion on some of the characters used in speciation of the genus. Mycopath. Mycol. appl. 33: 56-64.

Srivastava, R.C. 1976. Studies on fungi associated with fish diseases. Ph.D. Thesis, University of Gorakhpur, India. 101 pp.

Srivastava, R.C., and G.C. Srivastava. 1977. *Achlya caroliniana* Coker—a new record from India. Curr. Sci. 46: 422.

Srivastava, G.C., and R.C. Srivastava. 1977a. Host range of *Achlya prolifera* (Nees) de Bary on certain fresh water teleosts. Mycopathologia 61: 61-62.

Srivastava, G.C., and R.C. Srivastava. 1977b. *Dictyuchus anomalous* (Nagai), a new pathogen of fresh water teleosts. Curr. Sci. 46: 118.

Srivastava, G.C., and R.C. Srivastava. 1977c. Host range of *Saprolegnia ferax* (Gruith.) Thuret on certain fresh water teleosts. Curr. Sci. 46: 87.

Stafleu et al., ed. 1972. International Code of Botanical Nomenclature adopted by the Eleventh International Botanical Congress, Seattle, August 1969. Int. Bur. Plant Taxonomy and Nomenclature, Utrecht, Reg. veg. 82: 1-426.

Steffens, W., U. Lieder, D. Nehring and H.W. Hattop. 1961. Möglichkeiten and Gefahren der Anwendung von Malchitgrün in der Fischerei. Z. Fisch. 10: 745-771.

Stevens, R.B., ed. 1974. Mycology guidebook. University of Washington Press, Seattle. 703 pp.

Stevenson, A.B. 1970. Scourge of the salmon. New Scient. 45(689): 353, 354.

Stirling, A.B. 1879-1880. Additional observations on fungus disease of salmon and other fish. Proc. R. Soc. Edinb. 10: 371-378.

Stolk, A. 1958, Pathological parthenogenesis in viviparous toothcarps. Nature, Lond. 181: 1660.

Stolk, A. 1959. Development of ovarial teratomas in viviparous toothcarps by pathological parthenogenesis. Nature, Lond. 183: 763, 764.

Stolk, A. 1961. Pathological parthenogenesis in a viviparous toothcarp. Nature, Lond. 191: 507.

Strickland, K.L., and J.T. Carbery. 1968. Ulcerative dermal necrosis (UDN) of salmon in Ireland. Riv. ital. Piscic. Ittiop. 3: 12-15.

Stuart, M.R., and H.T. Fuller. 1968. Mycological aspects of diseased Atlantic salmon. Nature, Lond. 217: 90-92.

Sutton, B.C. 1973. Coelomycetes. Pages 513-582, in G.C. Ainsworth, F.K. Sparrow, and A.S. Sussman, eds., The fungi: an advanced treatise. Vol. 4A. Academic Press, New York.

Suzuki, S. 1960a. The seasonal variation of aquatic Phycomycetes in Lake Nakanuma. Jap. J. Ecol. 10: 215-218.

Suzuki, S. 1960b. Seasonal variation in the amount of zoospore of aquatic Phycomycetes in Lake Shinseiko. Bot. Mag., Tokyo 73: 483-486.

Suzuki, S., and H. Hatakeyama. 1961. Ecological studies of the aquatic fungi in Lake Yamanakako. Jap. J. Ecol. 11: 173-175.

Swarczewsky, B. 1914. Über den Lebencyclus einiger Haplosporidien. Arch. Protistenk. 33: 49-108, pls. 4-8.

Szaniszlo, P.J. 1965. A study of the effect of light and temperature on the formation of oögonia and oöspheres in *Saprolegnia diclina*. J. Elisha Mitchell scient. Soc. 81: 10-15.

Tack, E. 1960. Beiträge zur Erforschung der Forellen-Seuche. Allg. FischZtg 85: 634-635.

Tesarcík, J., and J. Hoska. 1962. Plísnová nákaza zaber síha severního marény. Veterinárství 2: 63-64.

Tesarcík, J., and Smísek, and K. Hluzek. 1965. Plísnová nákaza zaber síha severního marény. Veterinárství 3: 320-322.

Tiffney, W.N. 1939a. The identity of certain species of the Saprolegniaceae parasitic to fish. J. Elisha Mitchell scient. Soc. 55: 134-151.

Tiffney, W.N. 1939b. The host range of *Saprolegnia parasitica*. Mycologia 31: 310-321.

Tiffney, W.N., and F.T. Wolf. 1937. *Achlya flagellata* as a fish parasite. J. Elisha Mitchell scient. Soc. 53: 298-300.

Tománek, J. 1962. Plísnová nákaza zaber pstruhu duhových. Cslké. Ryb. 3: 36.

Triplett, E., and J.R. Calaprice. 1974. Changes in plasma constituents during spawning migration of Pacific salmons. J. Fish. Res. Bd Can. 31: 11-14.

Unger, F. 1844. Sur l'*Achlya prolifera*. Annls Sci. Nat., 3e sér., Bot., 2: 5-20.

Utida, S., T. Hirano, H. Oide, M. Ando, D.W. Johnson, and H.A. Bern. 1972. Hormonal control of the intestine and urinary bladder in teleost osmoregulation. Gen. comp. Endocr. Suppl. 3: 317-327.

Valéry-Mayet. 1885. Hatching salmon eggs at Montpellier, France, and trouble with fungus. Bull. U.S. Fish Comm. 5: 272.

Verdun, M. 1903. Mycose rénale chez une carpe commune. C.r. Séanc. Soc. Biol. 55: 1313-1314.

Vincent, E. 1908. Causes of disease in young salmonids. Bull. U.S. Bur. Fish. 28: 907-916 (issued August 1910).

Vishniac, H.S., and R.F. Nigrelli. 1957. The ability of the Saprolegniaceae to parasitize platyfish. Zoologica 42: 131-134.

Volf, F. 1933. Ein Beitrag zur Kenntis des Kiemenpilzes—*Branchiomyces sanguinis* (Plehn). Recl. Trav. Inst. Rechs. agron. Rép. Tchéc. 114: 2-13.

Volf, F. 1956. První záznam plísnové nákazy zaber u stik v nasich vodách. Sb. csl. Akad. zemed. Ved., Rada E, Zivocisná výroba 1:15-20.

Volz, P.A., and E.S. Beneke. 1972. A preliminary study of fresh water fungi from Abaco Island, the Bahamas. Mycopath. Mycol. appl. 46: 1-3.

Wachs, B. 1973. Bei Bachforellen experimentell erzeugte Symptome der geschwürigen Hautnekrose (UDN). Z. Wass. AbwasserForsch. 6: 153-159.

Walentowicz, A. 1885. Karpfenpest in Kaniow. Öst. Vjschr. wiss. VetKoe. 64: 193-200.

Walker, R. 1951. Mycetoma in a landlocked salmon. Anat. Rec. 111: 531. (Abstr.).

Waterhouse, G.M. 1973a. Peronosporales. Pages 165-183, *in* G.C. Ainsworth, F.K. Sparrow, and A.S. Sussman, eds. The Fungi: an advanced treatise. Vol. 4B. Academic Press, New York.

Waterhouse, G.M. 1973b. Entomophthorales. Pages 219-229, *in* G.C. Ainsworth, F.K. Sparrow, and A.S. Sussman, eds., The fungi: an advanced treatise. Vol. 4B. Academic Press, New York.

Webster, J. 1970. Introduction to fungi. Cambridge University Press, London. 424 pp.

Wedemeyer, G. 1969. Stress induced ascorbic acid depletion and cortisol production in two salmonid fishes. Comp. Biochem. Physiol. 29: 1247-1251.

Wedemeyer, G. 1970. The role of stress in disease resistance of fishes. Am.

Fish. Soc., Spec. Publ. 5: 30-35.
Wedemeyer, G.A., F.P. Meyer, and L. Smith. 1976. Environmental stress and fish diseases. Book 5 *in* S.F. Snieszko and H.R. Axelrod, eds., Diseases of fishes. T.F.H. Publications, Neptune City, N.J. 192 pp.
White, D.A. 1975. Ecology of an annual *Saprolegnia* sp. (Phycomycete) outbreak in wild brown trout. Verh. int. Verein. theor. angew. Limnol. 19: 2456-2460.
Willoughby, L.G. 1968. Atlantic salmon disease fungus. Nature, Lond. 217: 872-873.
Willoughby, L.G. 1969. Salmon disease in Windermere and the River Leven; the fungal aspect. Salm. Trout Mag. No. 186: 124-130.
Willoughby, L.G. 1970. Mycological aspects of a disease of young perch in Windermere. J. Fish Biol. 2: 113-116.
Willoughby, L.G. 1971. Observations on fungal parasites of Lake District salmonids. Salm. Trout Mag. No. 192: 152-158.
Willoughby, L.G. 1972. U.D.N. of Lake District trout and char: outward signs of infection and defense barriers examined further. Salm. Trout Mag. No. 195: 149-158.
Willoughby, L.G. 1977. An abbreviated life cycle in the salmonid fish *Saprolegnia*. Trans. Br. mycol. Soc. 69: 133-135.
Willoughby, L.G. 1978. Saprolegniasis of salmonid fish in Windermere: a critical analysis. J. Fish Dis. 1: 51-67.
Willoughby, L.G., and A.D. Pickering. 1977. Viable Saprolegniaceae spores on the epidermis of the salmonid fish *Salmo trutta* and *Salvelinus alpinus*. Trans. Br. mycol. Soc. 68: 91-95.
Wilson, J.G.M. 1976. Immunological aspects of fungal disease in fish. Pages 573-601, *in* E.B. Gareth Jones, ed., Recent advances in aquatic mycology. Paul Elek (Scientific Books) Ltd., London.
Winters, G.H. 1976. Recruitment mechanisms of southern Gulf of St. Lawrence Atlantic herring (*Clupea harengus harengus*). J. Fish. Res. Bd Can. 33: 1751-1763.
Witala, B., and M. Zielonka. 1974. Zgorzel skrzeli (branchiomycosis) u pstraga teczowego (*Salmo gairdneri* Rich.). Medycyna wet. 30: 603-605.
Wolf, F.T. 1939. Sawada's discovery of *Achlya flagellata* as a parasite of fish. Mycologia 31: 236-237.
Wolf, K. 1958. Fungus or *Saprolegnia* infestation of incubating fish eggs. Fishery Leafl. Fish Wildl. Serv. U.S. 460: 1-4.
Wolke, R.E. 1975. Pathology of bacterial and fungal diseases affecting fish. Pages 33-116, *in* W.E. Ribelin and G. Migaki, eds., The pathology of fishes. University of Wisconsin Press, Madison.
Wood, J.W. 1974. Diseases of Pacific salmon—their prevention and treatment, 2nd ed. Dept. Fish., Hatcheries Div., State of Washington. 82 pp.

Wood, E.M., W.T. Yasutake, and W.L. Lehman. 1955. A mycosis-like granuloma of fish. J. infect. Dis. 97: 262.

Woodhead, A.D. 1975. Endocrine physiology of fish migration. Oceanogr. mar. Biol. A. Rev. 13: 287-382.

Wundsch, H.H. 1929. Untersuchungen über die Kiemenfäule bei Fischen. II. Eine besondere Art der "Kiemenfäule" bei Hechten und Schleien. Z. Fisch. 27: 287-293.

Wundsch, H.H. 1930. Untersuchungen über die Kiemenfäule bei Fischen. III. Weitere Beobachtungen an *Branchiomyces demigrans* als Erreger der Kiemenfäule beim Hecht. Z. Fisch. 28: 391-402.

Wurmbach, H. 1951. Geschlechtunskehr bei Weibchen von *Lebistes reticulatus* Peters bei Befall mit *Ichthyophonus hoeri* Plehn-Mulsow. Wilhelm Roux Arch. EntwMech. Org. 145: 109-129.

Yang, B.-Y. 1962. *Basidiobolus meristosporus* of Taiwan. Taiwania 8: 17-27.

Young, N.A., K.J. Kwon-Chung, and J. Freeman. 1973. Subcutaneous abscess caused by *Phoma* sp. resembling *Pyrenochaeta romeror:* unique fungal infection occurring in immunosuppressed recipient of renal allograft. Am. J. clin. Pathol. 59: 810-816.

# Index

(Numbers within parentheses indicate pages with color illustrations; numbers in *italic type* indicate pages with either halftone illustrations or line drawings.)

— A —

*Achlya*, *10*, 12, 18
  morphological features of, *12*
  nomenclatural status of early records from fishes, 22
  species reported as fish parasites, 13-14
  zoospore development and release in *10* , *12*
*Achlya prolifera*, 14, 22
  confusions with *Saprolegnia ferax*, 21
*Aeromonas salmonicida*, 123
*Alburnus alburnus alborella* (bleak), 56
  branchiomycosis of, *53*, 55, (81, 84)
*Alosa pseudoharengus* (alewife), 87
*Amphiprion sebae* (yellowtailed anemonefish), 102
*Anabas testudineus* (climbing perch), 28
*Anguilla anguilla* (common eel), 56
*Anguilla japonica* (Japanese eel), 29, 37, 56
*Aphanomyces*, *10*, 12, 14
*Aphanopus carbo* (black scabbardfish), 87
Ascomycetes, 120-121
ascorbic acid metabolism of fish, 40
*Atherina boyeri* (Boyer's sand smelt), 56
*Aureobasidium*, 105-106
  as parasite of stingray (*Dasyatis*), *105*
  experimental infection of carp with, 106

— B —

*Bacillus Salmonis Pestis*, 21, 30
bacteria
  as cause of UDN, 30-31
  role of in "salmon disease", 21
*Basidiobolus* spp.
  as parasites of fishes, 62-63
Blastomycetes, 101, 102, 104
Bouin's fixative, 46
*Branchiomyces*, 50-60, *53*, (81, 84)
  culture of, 51
  host range and geographic distribution of, 54-57
  taxonomic problems with, 7, 51
*Branchiomyces demigrans*
  morphology and diagnostic features of, *52*

*Branchiomyces sanguinis*
  morphology and diagnostic features of, *52*
branchiomycosis
  chemoprophylaxis for, 60
  early studies of, 50
  environmental factors and prevention of, 59-60
  species of fishes susceptible to, 56-57
  symptoms of, 57-58

— C —

*Calyptralegnia*, *10*, 14
*Carassius auratus* (goldfish, wild goldfish), 22, 56, 103, 120
  saprolegniosis of, (68)
  *Verticillium* granuloma of, *116*
*Catastomus commersonii* (white sucker), 39
*Chondrostoma söetta* (Cyprinidae), 56
*Ciliata mustella* (fivebearded rockling), 61
*Cirrhinus mrigala* (Cyprinidae), 28
*Clupea harengus harengus* (Atlantic herring), 87
  experimental ichthyophonosis of, 98
  *Ichthyophonus* developmental cycle in, 64, 70-71, 74, 75, 98
  natural *Ichthyophonus* epizootics in, 98-99
*Cobitis taenia* (spined loach), 56
Coelomycetes, 116-119
coenocytic thallus, 9
*Colisa fasciata* (striped gourami), 28
*Colisa lalia* (dwarf gourami), 28
copper sulfate
  as algicide in fish ponds, 60
  treatment of branchiomycosis with, 59
*Coregonus albula* (European cisco), 56
*Coregonus* spp. (whitefishes), 22, 56
*Cottus asper* (prickly sculpin), 97
*Crenilabrus melops* (corkwing wrasse), 61
*Cyprinus carpio* (carp), 22, 56, 102
  *Basidiobolus* Infections of, 63
  branchiomycosis of, 50, (80, 81)
  *Dermocystidium cyprini* infections of, 124-125
  experimental ichthyophonosis of, 97
  *Fusarium culmorum* infections of, 111
  "Staff's disease" of, 45

155

## — D —

*Dermocystidium,* 122-126
  diagnostic features of species from Pacific salmon, (93, 96), 123-125
  pathology of, 124-125
  prevention and treatment of, 126
  probably not a fungus, 122-123
*Dictyuchus,* 10, 14

## — E —

*Erimyzon sucetta* (lake chubsucker), 28
*Esox lucius* (northern pike), 57
  branchiomycosis of, 50
*Esox niger* (chain pickerel), 29
*Exophiala,* 106-111
*Exophiala pisciphila*
  epizootic of channel catfish caused by, 110
  morphological and physiological features of, 107, 108
*Exophiala salmonis*
  histology of fishes infected with, 107
  morphological and physiological features of, 108
  symptoms of infection by, 106-107

## — F —

*Flexibacter columnaris,* 26
formalin
  as fixative, 46
  treatment of saprolegniosis with, 48
*Fundulus heteroclitus* (mummichog), 29, 102, 110
Fungi Imperfecti, 101-116
  species reported as fish parasites, 102-103
*Fusarium culmorum,* as parasite of carp, 111

## — G —

*Gadus morhua* (Atlantic cod), 87, 102
  *Exophiala* infections of, 110-111
  ichthyophonosis of, 97
*Gasterosteus aculeatus* (three spine stickleback), 57
*Gobio gobio* (gudgeon), 56
Grocott's methanamine-silver stain, 45

## — H —

*Helostoma temmincki* (Anabantidae), 28
heterothallism, 18
*Hippocampus erectus* (lined seahorse), 102, 110
Hyphomycetes, 104-116
  in fish tumors and granulomas, 105
*Hypophthalmichthys molotrix* (silver carp), 58

## — I —

*Ichthyophonus,* 61-100
  a complex of organisms, 64, 86
  infections recorded from freshwater salmonids, 90
  mode of infection by, 97
  recorded infections from North Atlantic fishes, 87
  systematics of, 61-64
*Ichthyophonus gasterophilum,* 61-62
*Ichthyophonus hoferi*
  conflicting interpretations of developmental cycle of, 64-83, *70, 74, 78*
  culture of, 86, (88)
  infection experiments with, 98
  morphology of, *66, 67,* (85, 89)
  natural epizootics of, 98-99
  probably not a fungus, 7, 64
  taxonomic and nomenclatural history of, 61-64
ichthyophonosis
  histology of, 85, *95*
  prevention and treatment of, 100
  sites of infection in, 94
  symptoms of (84, 85), 91
  thiamine deficiency disease and, 62
*Ichthyosporidium ( = Ichthyophonus),* 61-62
*Ictalurus melas* (black bullhead), 57
*Ictalurus nebulosus* (brown bullhead), 29
*Ictalurus punctatus* (channel catfish), 103
  *Exophiala* infections of, 110
intestinal saprolegniosis, 26
*Isoachyla,* 14-15

## — L —

Lagenidiales, 9, 12
*Lepomis gibbosus* (pumpkinseed), 28, 56
*Lepomis macrochirus* (bluegill), 56
*Leptolegnia,* 10
Leptomitales, 9, 16
*Leptomitus, 10,* 26-27
*Leuciscus cephalus* (chub), 56
*Limanda ferruginea* (yellowtail flounder), 87
  ichthyophonosis of, *67,* (89), *95,* 99
*Liparis liparis* (sea snail), 61
*Loricaria parva* (whiptail loricaria), 120
*Lota lota* (burbot), 57, 62

## — M —

*Macrozoarces americanus* (ocean pout), 100
malachite green
  as treatment for saprolegniosis, 48, (80)
  branchiomycosis and, 59

*Melanogrammus aeglefinus* (haddock), 87
methylene blue
  as treatment for branchiomycosis, 59
*Micropterus dolomieui* (smallmouth bass), 56
*Micropterus salmoides* (largemouth bass), 28, 56
microsporidians, 100
*Mollienesia (Poecilia) latipinna* (sailfin molly), 29
*Morone americana* (white perch), 29
*Myoxocephalus octodecemspinosus* (longhorn sculpin), 87

— N —

*Notopterus chitala* (featherback), 29

— O —

*Ochroconis (Scolecobasidium)*, 111-115
*Ochroconis humicola*
  morphology of, *112*
  infection of coho salmon by, *113, 114*
  rainbow trout infected by, 113
*Ochroconis tshawytschae*, 115
*Oncorhynchus kisutch* (coho salmon), 29, (65, 77), 90, 103
  *Dermocystidium* infections of, 123
  *Ochroconis* infections of, 112, *113, 114*
  *Phoma herbarum* infections of, 116-119
  saprolegniosis of, (65, 77)
*Oncorhynchus nerka* (sockeye salmon), 90
  *Dermocystidium* infections of, 93, 96, 123
  saprolegniosis of, (69, 72)
*Oncorhynchus rhodurus* (amago salmon), 102
  *Candida sake* infection of, 104
  saprolegniosis of gut in, 26
*Oncorhynchus tshawytscha* (chinook salmon), (65), 90, 103
  *Dermocystidium* infections of, 123
  *Ochroconis* infections of, 115
  *Phoma herbarum* infections of, (89, 92), 116-119, *118*
  saprolegniosis of, (65)
Oomycetes
  characteristics of potentially parasitic genera, *10*, 12
  compared to other fungi, 9
  earliest record of as fish parasite, 9
  genera and species reported as fish parasites, 12, 13-16
  morphological features of, 9, *10*
  "salmon disease" and, 19-20
  taxonomy of, 9, 12
oogamy, 9
oogonia, 18
oospores, 18-19

— P —

*Penicillium piscium*, 120-121
*Perca flavescens* (yellow perch), 29
*Perca fluviatilis* (perch), 10, 25, 57
  experimental ichthyophonosis of, 97
periodic acid-Schiff stain, 46
Peronosporales, 9
*Phoma herbarum*, (89, 92), *117, 118*
  as a parasite of salmonids, 116
  experimental infections of chinook salmon with, *118*, 119
  symptoms of infections by, (89, 92), 118
*Platichthys flesus* (flounder), 87
*Pleuronectes platessa* (plaice), 87
*Poecilia reticulata* (guppy), 29
  experimental saprolegniosis of, 37, (68, 73, 76)
*Pollachius virens* (pollock), 87
polyplanetism, 12
*Pomoxis nigromaculatus* (black crappie), 28
*Pseudopleuronectes americanus* (winter flounder), 87, 102, 110
*Ptychocheilus oregonensis* (squawfish), 97
*Puntius sophore* (Cyprinidae), 28
*Pythiopsis*, 10, 15
*Pythium*, 10

— Q —

quicklime (CaO), and branchiomycosis, 60

— R —

*Rutilus pigus* (Cyprinidae), 56
*Rutilus rutilus* (roach), 9

— S —

*Salmo clarki* (cutthroat trout), 103
  *Exophiala* infections of, 106
*Salmo gairdneri* (rainbow trout), 29, 57, 90, 103
  histopathology of ichthyophonosis in, (85), 94, 95
  *Ichthyophonus* developmental cycle in, 64, 78-79, 82
  intestinal saprolegniosis of, 26
  *Ochroconis* infections of, 113, 114
  *Phoma herbarum* infections of, 116-119
  saprolegniosis in eggs of, 69
  symptoms of ichthyophonosis in, 91
*Salmo salar* (Atlantic salmon), 29, 103
  and UDN, 27, *30, 31*
  *Exophiala* infections of, 110
  "salmon disease" of 1877-1881 in, 19-21

*Salmo trutta* (brown trout, sea trout), 29, 57, 87, 90
"salmon disease", roles of bacteria and fungi, 19-21
*Salvelinus alpinus* (Arctic char), 57
*Salvelinus fontinalis* (brook trout), 22, 90
  *Ichthyophonus* developmental cycle in, 64, 78-79, 82
  saprolegniosis of the gut in, 26
*Salvelinus namaycush* (lake trout), 103
  *Exophiala* infections of, 106
*Saprolegnia*
  aplanetism in, *17, 18*
  life cycle, *11*
  morphology of parasitic strains, 33, *34*
  species reported as fish parasites, 15-16
  zoosporogenesis in, *10*, 12, 17, *44*
*Saprolegnia diclina*
  intestinal saprolegniosis caused by, 26
  Type I, and saprolegniosis, 32-33
  UDN and, 31-32
*Saprolegnia diclina—Saprolegnia parasitica* complex, 25
*Saprolegnia ferax*, 15, 20, 22
  confusions with *Achlya prolifera*, 21
  intestinal saprolegniosis and, 26
*Saprolegnia parasitica*, 23-26
  a nomen ambiguum, 25
  description of, 23
  early concept of species, 23
  modern concept of species, 23-24
  UDN and, 32
*Saprolegnia shikotsuensis*, 16, 25
Saprolegniaceae
  as "opportunistic" primary parasites, 35
  genetic relatedness of genera in, 18
  meiosis and sexual reproduction in, 18-19
  nomenclatural status of early isolates from fishes, 22
  UDN and, 31-32
  zoospore development and release in, *10*, 12, 17, 18, *44*
saprolegniosis, 19-49
  ascorbic acid metabolism of host and, 40
  associated with wounds and lesions, 37
  early records of, 19
  first study of in Pacific salmon, 26
  fish eggs and, 45, (69)
  fishes experimentally infected with, 28-29
  gross pathology of, 43, *44*, (65, 68, 69)
  historical outline of, 19-32
  host debilitation hypothesis to explain, 32, 35
  in intestinal tracts of fishes, 26
  infection experiments and, 35-37
  isolation and culture of parasites causing, 42-43

lack of host inflammatory response in, 47
low host tissue specificity in, 46
mucus production and, 37
nature and causes of, 32-42
pathogenic strain hypothesis to explain, 32-33
plasma corticosteroid levels and, 41
prevention and treatment of, 47-49, (80)
proteolytic enzymes in, 33
sites of infection in, 44-45, 65, 68, 76, 77
stress hypothesis to explain, 38-41
symptoms of, 43
"tail nipping" and, 45
temperature effects and, 44
*Scardinius erythrophthalmus* (rudd), 56
*Scolecobasidium* (= *Ochroconis)*, 111-115
*Scomber scombrus* (Atlantic mackerel), 87
  *Ichthyophonus* developmental cycle in, 64, 82-83
*Semotilus atromaculatus* (creek chub), 28
*Silurus glanis* (European catfish), 57
  treatment of branchiomycosis in, 59
sodium chloride
  and treatment of saprolegniosis, 49
  to control branchiomycosis, 59
"Staff's disease", 45
staining techniques, 45-46
*Stenotomus chrysops* (scup), 102, 110
stress
  fungal pathogenicity, corticosteroid levels, and, 38-41
  protein deficiency and, 39
  UDN and, 27
stressors, 39
*Symphysodon axelrodi* (discusfish), (88)


— T —

Taumelkrankheit, 90
*Tautogolabrus adspersus* (cunner), 102, 110
thiamine deficiency and ichthyophonosis, 91
*Thraustotheca*, *10*, 16
*Tilapia* sp. (Cichlidae), 28
*Tinca tinca* (tench), 57, 102
  branchiomycosis of, 50
  experimental ichthyophonosis of, 97
*Trygon* (*Dasyatis*) *pastinacea* (common stingray), 102, 105


— U —

UDN (Ulcerative Dermal Necrosis), 20, *30, 31,* 45
  epizootic of Atlantic salmon and, 27
  role of *Saprolegnia* in, 32
  viruses and, 27

— V —

*Verticillium piscis*, 103, 116

— X —

*Xanthichthys ringens* (sargassum triggerfish), 102, 110

*Xiphophorus helleri* (green swordtail), 29
   experimental saprolegniosis of, 37, (76)
*Xiphophorus maculatus* (southern platyfish), 29

— Z —

zoosporangia, 9, *10, 17,* 44